ABOUT BEN

A Novel

ROBERT M. REECE

Paperback ISBN: 978-0-9914-4240-9
B&N ISBN: 979-8-3314-8488-0
Ebook ISBN: 978-0-9914424-1-6

Cover design by Thomas Tafuri
Covers by Tom and Jenny Lutz, Impact Graphics

Dedicated to Dr. Carl Weihl, University of Cincinnati Professor of Pediatrics and director of medical student pediatric education, who instructed hundreds of medical students in the art of pediatrics

Also by Robert M. Reece

To Tell The Truth
Double Blind Double Cross
Strong Medicine
The Lewellyns from Vincennes

"Being a practicing doctor is a calling. It's not just a job or a way to make a living. It's a sense that you must do this. Sort of a religious experience. You just know."

—Abraham Levinson, M.D.

CONTENTS

Chapter 1

Ben Levinson, 1952

A thunderclap headache woke Ben from his deep sleep. His pajamas were drenched with sweat and he was burning hot. He groped his way to the toilet, his hand guided by the top of a chest of drawers to the bathroom doorknob. He rested his hands on the raised toilet seat while he peed. *What's going on?* he wondered. His foggy brain conjured up an alarming dream just before awakening—struggling to run, in slow motion through heavy quicksand, from a frightening apparition whose form was other-worldly and ill-defined.

Splashing cold water on his face, he sloughed off the confusion of the night, looked in the mirror for reassurance that he was alive. Yes, alive. But not himself. He touched his forehead, then searched for a thermometer in the cabinet, shook the mercury down and took his temperature: 101.8 degrees Fahrenheit.

Oh, no! I can't get sick. I have to make rounds at the hospital.

Looking at his watch, he saw that he was already late. He shuffled into his bedroom, quickly threw on some clothes, and frantically knocked on his parents' bedroom door.

"Dad, can you take me to the hospital?" he shouted at the closed door frantically. "I'm late for rounds and I'll be even later if I take the T."

"Hold on, I'll dress and meet you downstairs," Jacob called out, recognizing panic in his son's voice.

In a few minutes, Ben and Jacob were soon on a crowded Route 9. Boston Pediatric Hospital was not far away.

"Thanks Dad, I'll see you at dinner," Ben said as he rose with major effort from the car at the entrance to the Fenway Building. He made his way to the elevators and joined the group of students, residents, and the preceptor at the bedside of a boy admitted with fever and sore throat.

This boy's sore throat was not a run-of-the mill pharyngitis. He had diphtheria, confirmed by culture two days before, a rare clinical condition since diphtheria vaccine had nearly eliminated the disease. The students looking in the patient's mouth saw a throat covered by a thick, grayish membrane and pus. They returned his mask quickly to his face.

A minute later Dr. Woolhandler, the attending pediatrician and preceptor, looked at Ben. He could tell immediately that he was not well.

"Go down to the student health center," he said to Ben with urgency and authority. "Your flushed face tells me you have a fever. So, make tracks and get seen. Don't come back to rounds. I'll check with you later."

At the health center, after taking his temperature, Ellie Linehan, the on-duty nurse, asked him routine questions about how his illness began, who his contacts were, and then looked at his throat and ears. She listened to his chest for breath sounds. "Sounds like you have a heavy respiratory infection," she said. "But with this fever—it's now up to 103—you should go home to bed, take some fever meds, drink lots of fluids. Stay away from any patients. I'm gonna do a throat culture and give you some acetaminophen. If your throat culture comes back positive for strep, we'll put you on penicillin. But for now, just symptomatic treatment. Come back tomorrow. If your fever's gone and your culture's negative, we'll decide what to do with you," she said in a friendly tone. "If you still have fever, we'll have Dr. Weller see you." She swabbed his throat for the culture and said, "So get on outta here. Hope you feel better. Check back in the morning. We're here after 8."

Ben trudged to the Longwood T station a half mile from the hospital. He considered calling his mother but decided against it. *Don't want to worry her*, he thought. By the time he got home, he was exhausted and went directly to bed. Sophie heard him come in and followed him up the stairs.

"What's wrong, Benji?"

"Got a fever and a headache. Saw the health center nurse at the hospital."

"What did she tell you?"

"Probably just a cold. Took a throat culture and wants me back tomorrow. Right now, all I want to do is sleep."

"Can I bring you anything?" Sophie asked, trying not to betray her concern. "Do you think I ought to call Dr. Lane?"

"No, and no. I'll be fine," he said impatiently. He got into bed, pulling the covers up to his neck as chills began to shake his teeth. He turned over and was asleep at once. He slept most of the day. When he woke up, his chills and fever were gone, and he felt close to normal.

Sophie was listening for him to wake up. She came up, peeked into his room, saw that he was awake.

"How're you doing?" she said.

"Still kind of woozy."

"Hungry? I can bring you something."

"Yeah, how about some soup?"

In a few minutes, Sophie brought him a bowl of chicken soup. "Some call this Jewish penicillin," she laughed. He eagerly spooned it in and after polishing it off promptly went back to sleep.

The next morning Ben told himself and his parents that he was fine. Sophie looked at him, shook her head, and said, "Are you sure? You seemed really sick yesterday. Why don't you stay home today?"

Ben reassured her as best he could and headed to the hospital for rounds. Arriving on the floor where rounds were just beginning, Dr. Woolhandler saw him and quickly asked, "What did they tell you at the health center yesterday?"

"Probably URI. Got a throat culture and she sent me home. Told me to come back this morning."

"So, why are you here and not at the health center?"

"I feel fine today," Ben said. "Really."

"What the hell is wrong with you? Get your ass down to the health center and find out about your culture and get further instructions," he said, clearly irritated. "This should be a good learning experience for you as a patient and a future doctor. Especially if you're seeing patients. A sick doctor is no good to his patients."

Ben felt chastised and angry, with himself and Dr. Woolhandler. His rising anger reminded him of an old problem, his short fuse when he thought he was treated unfairly. When he was in high school, he'd gotten into a fight with a classmate named Gerald during gym class. Gerald have shoved him aside to get to a ball during a volleyball game. Ben was infuriated by this and laid into Gerald, aiming a punch at his jaw but missing, striking his shoulder instead. Ben ended up with a trip to the doctor, X-rays, a plaster cast for a broken bone in his hand, suspension from school for fighting, and a referral for counselling to get his anger under control. He benefited from the counselling, but always was easily angered by what he considered unfair treatment.

Still, Dr. Woolhandler didn't have to embarrass him in front of the others. He knew Woolhandler was right. He shouldn't have come to rounds. When he got to the health center, he was pleased that the same nurse, Ellie, was there.

"Welcome back," Ellie said. "You look a lot better. Let me take your temp." After a minute, she took the thermometer out of his mouth. "Normal today. Let me check on your culture." She went to the incubator and took the culture plate out. "No bugs growing. Need to look again tomorrow to be sure, but no penicillin for now. You still shouldn't see patients, though. Go on home and rest. See me tomorrow."

Ben was glad the culture was negative, but he admitted to himself that he didn't feel one hundred percent well. He still had a headache, and his body hurt all over. Sort of like flu, he thought. He called the nurses' station on the ward and left a message for Dr. Woolhandler that he was advised to go home. Soon he called Ben at home. Sophie answered and passed the phone to Ben when she heard who was calling.

"Well, we're done for today anyway," Dr. Woolhandler said. "Rest, take lots of fluids. Nothing important here for you to do. Stay home until you're cleared by the health center to return."

The next few days all Ben could do was sleep. His rotation on pediatrics would be over at the end of the week, then he had a week off between rotations. He hated not seeing pediatric patients now, but he knew there would be other opportunities.

He was about to begin his medicine rotation when muscle pain in his legs began. He massaged his legs, hoping this would help, but it only made his legs hurt more. His neck was stiff when he tried to touch his chin to his chest, a maneuver he'd been taught as a medical student to check for meningitis. Even though he had no fever, he knew he needed to see a doctor. This wasn't right.

Sophie took him back to the health center and insisted on coming with him. Ellie wasn't there today, so he had to tell another nurse what had transpired. She listened sympathetically, but when he told her about his leg pain and stiff neck, she said, "Dr. Weller must see you. I don't like the sound of your new symptoms. Stay here and I'll get him."

Sophie's heart sped up as she crossed and uncrossed her legs, fidgeting with her purse. Ben didn't like his new symptoms either. As a medical student he began imagining all the possibilities, none of them good. *Relax, you're jumping to conclusions. Wait until the doctor sees you.*

Then the memory of a patient named Timmy popped into his head, and he got even more anxious. *Did I always wash my hands after examining him? Did I handle his bedpan? Were there other patients who might have had subclinical cases of polio when I took care of Timmy?*

His concern about polio was not unrealistic. He knew that polio cases were rising, and its mode of transmission was now understood to be from the intestines, so-called fecal-oral spread.

The door to the exam room opened and a small man, probably in his forties, came in. He was soft-spoken and had a kind air about him. He introduced himself, sat down opposite Ben and Sophie.

"You're Ben's mother? You must be very proud of him."

"Right now, I'm more worried than proud. I hope you can tell us what's going on."

"I'll do my best," Dr. Weller said, as he reached out to Sophie's hand to comfort her.

"So, tell me what's going on with you," he said, looking at Ben.

He recounted what he'd told the nurse.

"You're a medical student, right?" Dr. Weller said. Ben nodded.

"Are you worried about any particular disease?"

He looked at Sophie, not wanting to upset her further, but decided he had to tell Dr. Weller everything.

"I took care of a boy on my pediatrics rotation who ended up in an iron lung, so, yes, I'm worried about polio," he said, realizing how Sophie was hanging on his every word. She twisted a handkerchief in her hands and quietly groaned. She knew another family in Brookline grappling with the diagnosis of polio. And she read the newspapers about more cases being reported.

"I understand. But there are several other things in the differential diagnosis we need to consider. I think the most efficient way to look for all possibilities is to admit you. How do you feel about coming into the hospital?"

Ben swallowed hard. "Scared."

"It's good that you can admit that you're scared. It is scary, particularly as a medical student who knows many possibilities. But we should take a 'wait and see' approach. Stay optimistic. You're young and healthy, and you'll have the best medical team possible. You're in good hands."

Dr. Weller turned to Sophie.

"How're you doing?" he said, knowing the answer.

"Oy, Jacob, my husband, he doesn't even know we're here. I think I really need to call him. Do you have a phone I can use?"

"Sure. Come into my office, call him from there."

Ben liked Dr. Weller. He hoped to be like him when he got through his training. *Just like Uncle Abraham, devoted to his patients above all else.*

When Sophie and Dr. Weller returned, he said to Ben, "We'll arrange a bed for you on 6 West. There's a great group of residents on that floor."

"Did you get ahold of Dad?" Ben asked Sophie.

"Yes, thank God. He's very worried about you and he'll be here as soon as he can. He just needs to finish up with a customer and he'll be right on his way."

Chapter 2

Sophie and Jacob Levinson

Ben was the only child of Jacob and Sophie Levinson, not by choice but by circumstances.

After profuse postpartum bleeding forced her doctors to perform an emergency hysterectomy, her inability to have more than one child was a source of deep sadness for them both. She became a doting and anxious mother.

Sophie, also an only child, was petite, had black hair, dark eyes and a "great figure," according to her husband Jacob. Sophie's parents had emigrated from Germany to Brazil in the late '20s, witnessing the rising tide of anti-Semitism in Germany. Jacob and Sophie, recently married, followed their example by leaving Germany shortly afterwards, but to Boston instead of South America.

Jacob repeatedly admonished Sophie that she should stop "spoiling" young Benji, but her compulsion to hover over him couldn't be curbed. Jacob, with his methodical and all-business demeanor, tried to convince Sophie that Ben was perfectly healthy, but her need to protect him was exacerbated by his asthma attacks during his early childhood. She never could have imagined the later threat.

Ben was most fortunate to have been born in 1929, in Boston. He was called Benji by his mother, Benjamin by his father and Ben by everyone else. Although the United States was in the depths of a worldwide economic downturn that would define economic depressions for ensuing generations, his father, Jacob Levinson, was a prosperous jeweler.

Despite the Depression, he now owned a successful jewelry showroom on Washington Street in Boston's Downtown Crossing and several branch stores in the suburbs. The Levinsons lived in a spacious home in Chestnut Hill and by all measures were solidly upper-middle class, completely assimilated into an American style of living.

Ben grew to be taller than either of his parents, topping out at an even six feet. With black hair and eyes the color of teak set wide apart above a patrician nose, he became a person attracting attention from both sexes. His lanky frame was well-suited to his favorite sport of track, and he was liked by all who knew him. Now in his third year at Channing Medical School, he was delighted finally to be seeing real live patients.

On his pediatric rotation at Boston Pediatric Hospital, he assisted the residents in caring for several hospitalized children and kids in the outpatient clinics.

One was Timmy, a twelve-year-old Irish boy from Dorchester. He first met him in the Emergency Room, almost an afterthought in the building of inpatient services, a tiny corner in the domed Fenway building. Timmy came into the ER with a fever of 102 degrees, malaise, runny nose, wheezing, and headache. Most of these symptoms were run-of-the mill complaints, and after taking a history and doing an examination, Ben and his preceptor concluded he only had a cold with mild asthmatic bronchitis. They gave Timmy's mother instructions to give him plenty of fluids and treat any fever he had with some aspirin. They reassured her his wheezing would abate when the other symptoms cleared and sent them on their way.

But about a week later, Timmy returned to the ER. His headache had persisted, and he'd developed a stiff neck along with muscle weakness of his lower extremities. His wheezing, which was the symptom Timmy's mother feared most, had cleared, but these other symptoms prompted the medical staff to admit him to the inpatient service. Dr. Haynes, Ben's preceptor, assigned Timmy to him for a medical student workup.

Ben immediately took to Timmy, with his tousled reddish-auburn hair and bright blue eyes that sparkled with his quick wit and playful demeanor.

"Hey, Dr. Ben, ya know how a pilot likes his sandwich?" Timmy asked Ben during morning rounds by the medical team.

"No," replied Ben, as he cast a glance at Dr. Haynes, his preceptor, slightly embarrassed by Timmy's attention.

"Plane," Timmy said, giggling.

"What did the baby corn say to the mama corn?" Ben countered, as he now could see that Dr. Haynes was enjoying the banter.

"I give up," Timmy said with a broad grin on his face.

"Where's Popcorn?"

Because these silly jokes tickled everyone on rounds, they became a regular routine each day the "whitecoats" came by.

But Timmy's medical problem was no joke. It turned out to be the forerunner of the cascading endemic disease people all over the world morbidly feared in the early fifties.

Ben watched helplessly as Timmy's disease progressed from initial fevers and flaccid legs to assisted ventilation in an "iron lung." This life-preserving but frightening device was a metal cylinder with a tight-fitting opening for the patient's head at one end and a soft mattress inside. It worked by positive pressure cycling, forcing a patient's chest to mimic respiratory excursions.

Ben's initial thrill of taking care of patients turned to dark sadness as he watched Timmy become fully dependent on the ventilator. He would not leave this horrid -- but for some a lifesaving refuge -- until the end of his life when his other bodily systems failed. Other patients followed Timmy's fate as 1952 became one of the most disastrous years for polio. Ben was devastated by his death.

But that was not the worst of it for Ben.

Chapter 3

Uncle Abraham

When his father arrived, Ben was already on Six West in a private room. Jacob got into a gown and put on a mask and gloves just as Sophie and Dr. Weller had done.

"We've admitted Ben to do further testing, done more efficiently in the hospital," the doctor explained to Jacob. "He's not seriously ill, but we're extra careful with staff. They're exposed to so many different things. He looks fine. You're welcome to visit him whenever you'd like. I'm glad to answer any questions you have, now or anytime."

Jumping in, Sophie asked Dr. Weller, "What does he have?" She could barely get the words out.

"Undetermined right now. But with his history of fever, stiff neck and now muscle pain, we're doing a thorough workup."

Sophie sat down quickly on a chair, lightheadedness causing her balance to give way. Sophie was inherently anxious, unable to calm herself. She grabbed Jacob's hand and began to weep. Jacob, always the stabilizing force in their marriage, squeezed Sophie's hand and wiped away her tears. Jacob was just beginning to have a mid-waist bulge, but otherwise maintained his slender build. His full head of wavy hair was mixed gray and black, combed straight back from his high forehead. Sophie studied his barely lined middle-aged face for reassurance.

"Can I stay here overnight with him?" Sophie asked Dr. Weller.

"Wish I could say yes, but, sorry, hospital protocol won't allow that since he's in isolation. We don't want you exposed to any micro-organisms. Right now, we don't know what we're dealing with."

"Mom, try not to worry. These are top-notch doctors and nurses. They're taking good care of me." Ben did his best to project a hopeful demeanor.

"Have they told you what's wrong, what you have?" Sophie asked.

"It's early, Mom, that's why I'm here, to find out what this is."

"What are they thinking about?" she persisted, knowing, in her heart what they were looking for, having heard Benji describe his experience of taking care of Timmy.

"If anyone could answer that question, it would be the doctors. They're looking at all the possibilities."

"Such as?" Sophie pressed on. It was odd, but she seemed to want to hear the dreaded word "polio." Perhaps she wanted to be sure the doctors were considering this, which on reflection she knew was ridiculous.

"Well," Ben began patiently, "I'm only a medical student, but since this began as a fever, I'd say they're looking for an infection, taking cultures, watching me for other possibilities. They're factoring in what other kinds of cases are in the hospital, especially patients I've seen, been exposed to."

"You know what's being said in the papers, don't you?" Sophie said, too upset herself to consider that her fretting might be raising Ben's anxiety.

"Yeah, sure, of course I know what's in the news. But what makes newspaper headlines is not how diagnoses are made. They're approaching this the right way," Ben said, trying to reassure Sophie, and himself, at the same time.

"I'm sure they're doing their best," Jacob finally said, trying to display calm. "In the meantime, we mustn't jump to conclusions. Need to take this day to day." Jacob, ever the rational voice, was trying to keep his own panic under control.

The next day was a marathon of tests and consultations, with a sea of faces congregating around Ben's bed. Being the center of so much attention made him even more anxious. Some of his fellow medical students came to see him, all required to wear facemasks, gloves, and surgical gowns before entering his room, so it was hard for him to recognize most of them. He greeted them as though this were a social call, trying to be more reassuring to them than they could be to him. There was an abundance of laughter and bonhomie, but everyone knew that something serious was up. They also knew what they'd been seeing in patients at Boston Pediatrics Hospital--poliomyelitis.

Dr. Weller came by after the medical students left.

"Hi Ben. How're you feeling?" Not waiting for an answer, he said, "I need to do a lumbar puncture to get some spinal fluid for analysis. You know how it's done. You lie on your left side, a little Novocain around the site. Your job is to make like a cat on a hot tin roof making your back curve outward so I can slip the needle in smoothly. It'll be over before you can say 'Jack Robinson.' "

"I've done these," Ben said. "I hope you're better at it than I am," remembering a time when he struggled to get the needle into the right place in the spinal canal of a two-month-old infant.

"I've done this on hundreds in kids much smaller than you, who tend to squirm around. Yours should be easy."

The spinal tap went well and when he returned from the treatment room he promptly went to sleep. Within minutes, he was awakened from sleep by a familiar voice.

"How is my favorite nephew?" Abraham said as soon as he sat down.

"Uncle Abraham! How are you? Thanks for coming to see me," Ben said, perking up. "Well, I guess I've seen better days."

"I came as soon as I heard. Is there anything I can do for you?"

"Tell me what you think I've got."

"What do you think you've got?" Abraham replied, answering Ben's question with a question, in true physician mode.

"It looks to me like polio. Why am I getting this as an adult? I thought this was a kid's disease, you know, infantile paralysis."

"Fewer infants get this than older children. And adults get it too. You, of course, know about Roosevelt. Some doctors think he had Guillain-Barre syndrome, but most think he had polio because his paralysis never disappeared. In Guillain-Barre the paralysis most often fades away. Roosevelt's polio case was a rarity. A very small percentage of polio cases get paralysis.

"Did you treat anyone recently with polio?" Abraham asked.

"Well, yeah, a kid named Timmy. He had an awful case. Spent his last days in an iron lung. And I probably saw others who didn't get as sick. From what I hear, new records are being set this year in the number of cases." His eyes fixed on Abraham. "But don't tell Mom if you think this is polio. She's going bonkers worrying. If the doctors conclude it's polio, we'll obviously need to tell her, but 'til then I don't want her to have to face reality. It'll take her time to adjust to the idea." He paused, then said, "It'll take me some time, too."

"My guess is that your mother knows already," Jacob said quietly. "She has a generous amount of intuition."

Just then, the nurse came into the room to make evening rounds. "Sorry to interrupt, but anything you need before it's lights out?"

"No, thanks," Ben said. Pointing to his uncle, he said. "This is my uncle, Dr. Abraham Levinson. He works at MIT."

"Pleased to meet you, sir. What kind of doctor are you?"

"Medical doctor. I was an old-fashioned GP, but now I do research," Abraham replied.

"Glad to meet you, sir. Being a doctor seems to run in your family, Ben," she said as she left.

"I must leave now," Abraham said, betraying only a slight German accent but speaking in formal English. "I will come to see you in a week or so. I am going to New York for a project I am working on. I won't be back until next Thursday. I might be able to come here on Friday. By that time, you might even be home. I hope so.

"I love you, Ben. You will be in my prayers until we meet again."

~~~
~~~

Seeing his favorite uncle reawakened intense memories of Abraham's surprise arrival into their family's life years earlier. His father, one night at dinner, announced to the family, "I just got a letter from my brother, Abraham." He paused, trying to gauge Sophie's reaction to this sudden news from his hitherto uncommunicative brother. "He's coming here from Canada, a country he was somehow able to get in from Germany. He has no job and no money." Jacob looked at Sophie again. "We've got to take him in."

Sophie stared at Jacob, hand on forehead, her fork raised halfway to her mouth. "What do you mean, we've got to take him in?" was all she could say, astounded by this unexpected declaration. "Do you mean to this house?"

"Yes."

"When?"

"I don't know exactly, he didn't say. Soon. Um, I think he could stay in our spare bedroom until he gets oriented and back on his feet. His letter was succinct, ah, you might even say abrupt. You know I haven't heard from him in years, maybe due to, shall we say, the unsettled politics over there."

Sophie's mind was gyrating wildly. She never understood the reasons that Jacob and Abraham had never been close, one could even say alienated. But Sophie understood there was no way she could object to his coming. He was family, after all, and the world situation so dire, especially in Germany, that not to take him in would be horribly insensitive, to say nothing of her strong belief in family loyalty. Jacob and Sophie both understood they had no choice.

"Do you know what his mental state is? He lost his wife recently, didn't he? And were there children?" Sophie asked.

"I think he's quite alone," Jacob said. "He had no children. He's never been an easy person, you know. He was blindly devoted to his medical practice to the exclusion of everything else."

Jacob had kept track of events in his native Germany in 1939. He'd read reports that Germany was descending into an absolute dictatorship under Hitler with deeper anti-Semitism than ever. Dark rumors had reached the United States of Jews being rounded up and forced into concentration camps after the infamous Kristallnacht horror of October 1938. He'd read the news about that night, when anti-Semitic zealots, encouraged by the Nazi government and Hitler himself, destroyed 267 synagogues and over 7,000 Jewish businesses in Germany, Austria, and Sudetenland. The estimate of Jewish fatalities was in the hundreds. Abraham's escape from Hamburg was a miracle. It would be a subject Jacob hoped to learn more about once he was settled.

Jacob and Sophie had left Germany eleven years before, when Jacob recognized then that the political path was veering sharply toward totalitarianism. He'd told Sophie at the time, "I think it's time to leave."

Sophie and Jacob could, without guilt but with much regret, leave the country of their birth.

Jacob had built a successful jewelry business in Germany and was able to sell it at a handsome profit before the depression had begun. When he came to Boston, he was fortunate to find a jewelry business for sale. He and Sophie both wanted desperately to assimilate into their new country. They had studied English in German schools and, with several intense months of courses in conversational English in America, now spoke flawless American English. Their teacher said she had never seen students who picked up the accent and the idiom as quickly. Sophie was naturally outgoing and both she and Jacob quickly adopted American customs.

Ben had never met, nor even been aware of his Uncle Abraham, but he was told that he'd been a physician in Germany, taking care of the poor in Hamburg, which must have accounted for his current lack of money. Jacob reasoned that he'd spent what meager savings he had for the trip to Canada and now had no alternative but to ask for help from his brother.

Jacob's relationship to him had always been distant. Abraham, who was ten years older, had a distinctly different temperament than his little brother. Jacob had always been interested in business and money-making, whereas Abraham had been dedicated to service in his community. From very early on, Jacob resented his older brother for what he considered his mother's partiality. He even referred to Abraham as "the most favored son" in the family. His entry into medical school solidified this charmed position and led to Jacob's resentment, jealousy, and ultimate rejection of his brother. Now he had to welcome him and give him a place to live.

For Ben, at age ten, Abraham's coming was an exciting event in his young life. To meet his German uncle, a doctor dedicated to caring for the poor, was exciting to Ben in an abstract way. He was too young to be an idealist, but Abraham seemed to be very unlike other adults he knew.

"What does he look like?" Ben asked.

"Well, he's ten years older than I, and I've not seen him in years," Jacob said. "He used to have a dense black beard, and he would go without haircuts for months, so preoccupied with his patients that he neglected everything else, even his wife. Why, I don't understand. I recall his wife as a sweet lady. Maybe we'll find out more when he gets here," Jacob said, avoiding an explanation that might suggest how impoverished was his real relationship with his brother.

Conversation paused as each of them tried to imagine what life would be like when this mysterious stranger began living with them.

"He must have been desperate to escape. To be stripped suddenly of his daily life, as ascetic as it must have been," Jacob said. "He had to be lonely, losing his wife and having no other family."

"If he hadn't gotten out of Germany, he could have been arrested and shipped off to those infamous camps." Sophie wondered aloud if these camps really existed. "Or were they just horror stories told among my Jewish friends?"

"From what I've read in the *New York Times*, these camps do exist and are truly barbaric," Jacob said.

"How could this fate befall our homeland?" she mused. "A place that produced Mozart, Beethoven, Goethe, and a host of artists and philosophers? All the great scientific discoveries in medicine, physics, engineering?"

Jacob just shook his head. Ben listened intently to this conversation, unaware of the conditions in his parent's country of origin. He didn't ask what his father meant by "barbaric," but he'd heard stories from his classmates who had relatives in Germany.

Jacob couldn't fathom how Abraham managed to get out of Germany when every exit seemed to be blocked to Jews. He didn't know how well he spoke English.

The following Sunday Abraham surprised Jacob with a telephone call.

"Jacob, this is Abraham," he said with only a slight German accent, satisfying Jacob's wondering about his fluency in English. "I'm in Boston at the bus station downtown. I'm terribly sorry to be such a burden to you, but I have no choice. Would it be possible for you to pick me up?"

Astonished by the surprise call, Jacob could only say, "Abraham! I can hardly wait to see you! It's been so long since we've heard from you. We're so horrified at what's happening in Germany. It's such a relief to hear from you. How are you?"

"I'm tired, hungry, and nervous, but otherwise fine."

"Of course, I'll pick you up! Go to the front entrance of the station and look for a dark green sedan. My son Ben will be with me. He's so eager to meet you," Jacob said hurriedly. "How will I know you? What are you wearing?"

"A black suit, white shirt, and blue tie," he said. After a few anxious seconds he asked, "How long will it take you to get here?"

"Depending on traffic, about thirty minutes. See you soon!"

Jacob went to tell Sophie and called Ben from the backyard where he was playing toss with Slocum, his black Lab.

"Sophie, I'll take Ben with me to pick him up. Do you want to come?"

"No, I need to stay here, make sure I've got the room ready for him. What do you think I should make for dinner?"

"I'm sure he'd like chicken in the pot, some mashed potatoes, some kind of greens. I don't know what he likes to drink. We'll find out when he gets here."

They were all excited, Ben recalled. He thought his mother was mostly nervous, but she was a good cook, he knew that. Jacob and Ben jumped into the car and headed downtown to meet the enigmatic Dr. Abraham Levinson.

Ben was abruptly jerked back into the present by a nurse who came into his room to check his vital signs. He came out of his reverie, having remembered with amazing clarity the events of his uncle's arrival. Those had been exciting days for a ten-year-old.

~~~

In the morning of his tenth hospital day, Ben tried to get out of bed to go to the toilet, but his legs wouldn't respond. Try as he might, he couldn't move them. He reached down and pushed his right leg to the edge of the bed, then the left. He sat up, using his upper body strength, but still couldn't move his legs. He pressed the call button on his bed.

"You called?" said June, the nurse who came in.

"I was getting up to go to the bathroom to pee, but I can't move my legs. I have to go badly."

She listened, looked at him with concern, and said, "Lie back down, I'll get a urinal for you, and call the resident. Don't try to get out of bed. I'll be right back."

Ben then knew what he had.
~~~

Chapter 4

Arlene

June returned, gloved, masked and in a gown. She handed a cold metal urinal to Ben and after assuring herself that he was stable on the edge of the bed, she left his room. He reached down and positioned the urinal, shuddering at the chill of the metal against the skin of his thighs. He sat there expecting to urinate quickly, but nothing happened. His bladder was uncomfortably full, but he simply couldn't get a flow started.

Dammit, my sphincter muscle must be paralyzed too, he thought, remembering his freshman anatomy course. As he absorbed this reality, his mood darkened. *Am I gonna live like this forever? Am I even going to live, or die like Timmy?*

"Can I take that from you now?" June asked gently when she returned, seeing that Ben was still holding the urinal under his hospital gown. He slid it out and handed the empty vessel to her.

"I couldn't pee. Leave it here, maybe I can later," he mumbled, disconsolate with his failure of control.

"Sure," she said, understanding his embarrassment. "I'll put it right here on your nightstand." Turning toward him, she said, "Can I help you lie down now?"

"Yeah. But I'm really uncomfortable. I can feel my bladder's extra full. Can you get someone to help me with that?"

"I've already called the resident. He should be here soon."

I wonder if the same thing will happen when I need to poop, he thought, his gloom becoming darker by the minute.

"This is miserable. Why is this happening to me? I've done nothing to deserve this," Ben said aloud to no one, channeling everyone who has suffered profound trauma.

The resident, a young man Ben remembered seeing around the hospital, came in with the catheter kit wrapped in a blue cotton sterilized pack. He waved to Ben, smiled, and said,

"I'm Paul Garrett, urology resident on call. You know why I'm here, right?" To try and assure Ben of his competence, he said, "Don't worry, I've done a whole lot of catheterizations. Have you ever been cathed before?"

"Nope. Never needed it 'til now."

Paul explained the process, which Ben already knew, pulled on his rubber gloves, prepped Ben with an antiseptic, and slipped the lubricated catheter in. The procedure was over in short order.

After he was done, he held the collecting container up and told Ben, "1100 milliliters of urine. No wonder you were uncomfortable. I'll send this to the lab, but it looks clear."

"Thanks, Paul. I hope I never see you again," Ben said, smiling at his own gallows humor. "No offense."

"None taken, but if you need another cath, I won't take it out on you," Paul said, joining Ben in the ribbing.

Ben looked around his room. Typical hospital room, green walls, linoleum tile floor, high plaster ceiling with exposed plumbing pipes. On the wall were dangling blood pressure cuffs, otoscopes, oxygen outlets, and other medical paraphernalia. On the foot of his bed hung a clipboard with a line of scribbles indicating his vital signs over time. His complete hospital medical record containing more detailed clinical information was in a hinged stainless-steel cover, suspended with the other patient's chart in a bulky and noisy chart rack on wheels that residents pushed ahead of them on rounds. Ben gradually accepted an obvious and stark reality: being a patient was an entirely different experience than being a doctor or nurse. This was the other side of the contract between doctor and patient. He'd never been in this role in a hospital.

After a few minutes, the door opened again, and a young woman approached his bed.

"Hi Mr. Levinson, I'm Arlene Williams. From physical therapy. How're you doing?" Her dark hair was cropped short, there were some faint crow's feet around her blue eyes. Because she was masked and wearing a gown, Ben could tell little about the rest of her.

"Hello," Ben said tentatively, not knowing what she was here to do.

"The nurse told me you're not able to move your legs. I'll try to help with that," she said, almost reading his mind. "I'll be working with you to strengthen those muscles and try to get you moving again."

"Yeah. Just seemed to happen overnight. I was fine when I went to sleep last night. The other thing is pain, a lot of pain in my legs."

"I saw in your chart you're a medical student. So, you must be aware of your diagnosis, right?"

"Yeah," he answered, looking at the floor. He hesitated for a moment. "Maybe you can answer a question for me"

"I'll try."

"I just had to be cathed. In addition to my useless and painful legs, I also can't urinate. Can I expect to be unable to move my bowels too? I'm worried about this."

"Those two things can go together, but they often correct themselves," she said, looking directly at Ben.

"So, as a med student you may remember that paralysis of the lower limbs from polio is due to destruction of motor neurons in the spinal cord below a certain level. Lower extremity paralysis in polio is usually just on one side, but not always. It's often transient, too, so physical therapy is best begun early. The other thing to remember is that neuronal destruction in polio is spotty and what's true today may not be true tomorrow. So, in answer to your question: we'll be watching and waiting to see how it develops.

"I'm here to work with you to keep your leg muscles moving so they don't lose tone," Arlene continued. "Movement is the best way to accomplish that. There have been some recent papers that suggest that warm compresses help arrest the paralysis or at least mitigate it. Ever hear of Sister Kenny?"

"Uh, no, she a nun or something?"

"No, not sure why she's called Sister Kenny. She's not a nun, but she's gained fame for using warm compresses and massage to alter the course of polio paralysis. She's very influential, and her approach has been adopted in many places. So, after I evaluate you, we can start on this regimen. OK?"

"OK. Have at it," Ben said, trying to project optimism.

Arlene brought in her cart and had Ben lie down. She applied steaming towels to his legs from the thighs to the ankles. He grimaced when she first touched his sensitive legs, but they began to feel better as the packs stayed on. The thought that therapy with such dispatch gave him hope. Later he learned that Sister Kenny's therapy was found to be of little use in restoring function. The upside of her therapy was that it did no harm and made patients feel better, knowing that something was being done for them.

After the towels had cooled, Arlene removed them and rolled a walker to the bed.

"Can you sit up on the edge of the bed?"

Ben pushed up with his hands, then used them to move his legs between the upright legs of the walker. He grimaced as he fought to control the pain.

"Now I'm going to support you as you ever so slowly stand up. Put your weight on your hands and forearms as you grasp the handles. We'll see if we can make this work. The first time is always a little tricky, so take it slow and easy."

With his legs dropped between the vertical legs of the walker and with the weight of his torso transferred onto his arms, Ben was able to assume an upright position. But he still couldn't move his legs, and they wouldn't support his upper body. Arlene was still holding him up with an arm around his waist.

"Good work, Ben. Now sit back down. That's the first time and I don't want to push you too hard." Arlene knew that physical therapists had a reputation of driving people to perform beyond their capabilities. Some subscribed to the mantra "no pain, no gain." She was not of that school and Ben came to appreciate that. After she helped position him in bed, she said, "I'll see you tomorrow. We'll work together to get you going gradually. Can I get you anything before I leave?"

"Can you ask the nurse to bring my pain meds in?"

"Sure. Anything else?"

"Well, I'd like something new to read. Reading does distract me from the pain and my bad moods. I've finished several books and lying here without having something else to think about is, well, for want of a different word, depressing."

"How about if I have the nurses bring you today's Globe?"

"Great, I haven't seen a newspaper since this all started. I used to read the paper every day."

"I'm sure one of the nurses has a copy. I'll ask them."

Ben liked her. She was direct and clear in her approach without being harsh or patronizing. He was grateful to be in this hospital with many good hands caring for him.

Happy to get the Globe, he turned immediately to the sports section. News of his favorite team, the Boston Red Sox, was not good. Ted Williams, much to the dismay of all Red Sox fans, had been called back to military service, serving as a combat pilot in the Korean War. The team was languishing in last place. Teddy Ballgame, as he came to be known, had played in only six games before he departed. The hated

Yankees were riding high and were favored not only to win the American League championship, but the World Series again.

Looks like the Sox season is over, Ben thought. To add to the misery, Walt Dropo and Johnny Pesky were traded to Detroit and Jimmy Piersall was in a mental health facility because of his repeated out-of-control outbursts during games. It had not been a good season for the hometown team.

Ben turned to another page. "Raging Polio Epidemic in Copenhagen, Denmark, Rising Polio Threat in the US" were the headlines. There had also been a major spike in cases in Texas in April. The only good news about polio was that scientific work on a vaccine looked promising. But not in time to help him.

In other news, he read that Dwight Eisenhower, the Republican candidate for president, was busily campaigning against Adlai Stevenson, his Democrat opponent. All indications were that Eisenhower would win because of his reputation as the hero general of D-Day.

As he laid the paper down, his thoughts shifted to Franklin Delano Roosevelt. What Ben couldn't know was how seriously paralyzed he was. FDR and his handlers were adamant that his disease would not interfere with his performance as president. They downplayed the extent of his disability and FDR himself did his best to disguise it, struggling to a standing position with herculean help from his aides, but never betraying the amount of help he needed and the pain he endured by keeping up the pretense that his paralysis was not a problem. *What a courageous man,* Ben thought. *He must have been as pissed off as I am about getting this damned disease. There are days when I could scream out words that would shame a longshoreman.*

His thoughts turned to other possible consequences of his plight. *What if the medical school decides not to allow me to continue if I can't walk? Have there been other medical students who got sick making them less able to perform than when they began? Who can I talk to about this? Could all the hard work I've done to get into and perform in med school go down the drain? Will I ever be able to find a girl who'll have me, a cripple? Will I ever have kids?* He thought about Timmy again, how much he'd liked that kid. *Is there a God up there? What's going on, God? Why do you allow diseases like this to exist?* Then he began to make a mental list all the wrongs in the world.

Stop! he finally told himself. *Stop this whining! You're still alive and still have a functioning brain. You aren't blind, or deaf, or mute, and you don't have the ninety-seven other things that can happen to people. So, count your blessings.* He gradually calmed down and drifted into a semi-sleep, knowing he was going to need another catheter before the real night began.

Chapter 5

Cathy and Abraham

Ben saw the early light of a new day filter through the grime on his hospital window and wondered what challenges today would bring. *Would paralysis afflict other parts of his body? Would he end up in an iron lung like Timmy? Is it possible his bladder sphincter recovers so he wouldn't need repeated catheterizations?*

Thinking of which, one thing needed to be done immediately. He rang his buzzer for the nurse.

"Could you call Dr. Garrett to come and cath me again?" he asked a nurse he'd never seen before.

"Sure, glad to. Anything else?"

"Uh, no. But may I ask your name? I've not met you before."

"I'm Cathy. New to this floor. I've been working on the 8th floor, but they needed another nurse here. Things have gotten quite busy."

"What's the story? Why so busy?"

"Big influx of cases like yours. Seems we're in an epidemic."

"That's what I've heard. The newspapers say it's not only here, but in Europe as well," Ben said. "Are the cases here like mine with paralysis, or only fever, aches, and pains?" His clinical curiosity continued to be aroused, even as he was a victim of this epidemic.

"Most don't have any paralysis, thank heaven. But people are pretty sick." She examined his face. "I've seen you around. You're a medical student, right?"

"Yeah, third year. I can't tell if I've seen you before, what with the mask, gown, and hair covering. Have you been on pediatrics? I was there last rotation. That's where I must have picked this up."

"Yeah, I was on pediatrics."

Cathy stepped back from the bed, lowered her mask revealing full bow-shaped lips below a narrow straight nose, framed by high cheekbones. Ben had already noticed her green eyes, and her cap failed to cover a few wisps of dark brown hair. Ben felt a warm flush in his face and realized he was getting ruddy. He'd spotted her before on pediatric rounds and remembered he'd been struck by her beauty and had thought, *What a body!*

"Now I remember you, for sure," he said, trying not to betray that it was more than merely noticing her.

Seeing Ben's transparent reaction, Cathy felt obliged to get back to business quickly.

"I'll call the urology resident right away. See ya later," she said, more than a little self-conscious by his reaction to her "unveiling." She hurried out of the room.

After he'd been cathed, Arlene came back to work with him. She was more aggressive today and by the time she was finished, Ben was weary. He'd almost fallen asleep when a familiar voice roused him.

"Ben? Feel up to having a visitor?" Abraham said.

"Absolutely! You're always welcome, Uncle!" he cried out, quickly wide awake, so pleased that Abraham had come. "This is a great time. I've just been cathed and finished with PT. Come and sit down!"

"Just got in from New York and thought I'd stop by before I went home. So, how are you doing? What's with the catheter?"

"Have you talked with Mom and Dad?"

"No. I wanted to see you before I talked with them. Since you're still here, you must not be as well as when I left."

"My legs are paralyzed. And so are my sphincters," Ben said, speaking in staccato rhythm. "I'm getting PT, and I'm being cathed every six hours."

Abraham paused before responding, knowing these signs of pressured speech were indicative of Ben's agitated low spirits.

"How is your mood?" Abraham asked gently.

"As you can imagine, not good. But I'm not deeply depressed, if that's what you mean. Then again, my prospects are not all that great. How can I practice medicine, paralyzed? Having to be catheterized every six hours?"

"The first thing I can tell you is that your paralysis could be temporary. So might the sphincters problem.

"Secondly, if your paralysis does stay with you, modern equipment is now available to make it possible to do many things that before weren't possible. The other thing, I can't be sure of this, but the sphincter problems will likely go away."

Ben sighed and, wiping an unwelcome tear from his cheek, he said, "Looking ahead sure is different. All these complications.

"I won't be able to drive, for example. I only can go where there are elevators, I'll have to plan in detail for every little thing, needing help for almost everything," Ben was getting into a darker place as he contemplated his future. "No sex life, no girlfriends, people staring at me like I'm a freak."

"Ben, listen to me," he began, moving his chair closer to the bed and fixing him with his intense eyes. "Some of what you say is true. Things will be different. But your concern about girlfriends, sex life, people looking at you, not driving—that's fear talking. There are always paths around obstacles. You'll find those. You're very inventive. Your brain works as well as ever, you're young and otherwise healthy." Abraham took his hand in his. "You'll figure this out. Sophie and Jacob will help as long as you need them. And I'm around to pitch in."

This last statement really got to Ben. He began sobbing from deep inside. Abraham shot up from his seat and held Ben in his arms until he was able to get back in control.

Ben said, "Do you think they'll let me finish medical school?" His voice trembled as he asked the question that topped his worry list.

"I have no question about that," Abraham said firmly. "How could they not let you finish? The profession of medicine is wholly rooted in empathy, kindness, and a desire to help one's fellow men and women. The idea that they would throw you overboard is completely unwarranted, so put that out of your mind."

Once Ben was back in control, Abraham released his grip on his nephew and sat back down.

"Let me tell you a story," Abraham began. He knew that when Ben was young, he loved to hear stories about medical cases, ones that were about patients that would carry meanings.

"I once took care of a young man who had a ruptured aneurysm in his brain. This unexpected brain injury caused a right-sided paralysis, and it took him weeks to be able to do most of the things that most of us do without thinking.

"He was in love before the accident. But now he stubbornly refused to see his girlfriend; he didn't want her to see his incapacitation. She was devastated, but she kept trying to make him understand that she loved him, no matter what. He continued to push her away, but she persisted. One day, without warning, she came to his house where he lived with his parents. For the first time, she saw him in his wheelchair, unable to move his right arm and leg. He screamed repeatedly "You have to leave!" But she refused to leave, over and over, until he finally stopped yelling at her.

"I love you. That's all that matters," she said, tears rolling down her soft cheeks.

"That's the message here, Ben. Remember, love is independent of physical endowments, it is a felt entity springing from the spirit."

Ben had listened intently to his uncle as he related his story of devotion, then said, "What happened to them?" still skeptical that this had a happy ending.

"They later married and had several children. He found work helping others to find their way. I lost track of them when I came to America, but I want to believe they survived the war and raised their family."

Their conversation paused as both became contemplative, moving into those private spaces in the mind reserved for quiet.

After a few moments, Ben said, "Uncle, I've meant to ask you a couple of things since the day you arrived. One is how you learned to speak English so well, never having lived outside of Germany."

"That is easy to answer. I roomed with a fellow named Ken Monroe for four years in medical school. He was from St. Louis in Missouri, I think, and he taught me English as it is spoken in America. His accent and the way he talked has stuck with me ever since."

Ben was unsure of how to ask the other question he had, an even more sensitive one. "I hope you don't take this the wrong way, but I'm so curious about another thing, I can't help but ask. How did you tolerate the inhumanities you witnessed in Germany?"

"My patients needed me and that's all I allowed myself to think about. I also knew that resisting the political forces that were prevailing would do no good and only cause more oppression. When the war came, so many people were lost, so many died, large numbers of life records were destroyed or lost. The camps were everywhere." He looked out the window, his eyes unfocused. "I probably will never know what happened to many of my friends and patients. It's what I must live with. I have no choice."

Ben initially felt guilty for causing his uncle to reopen these wounds. But, as he pondered more, he rationalized his curiosity. He knew he'd become a surrogate son to his uncle, so perhaps his question would enable Abraham to talk about his losses with him when melancholy came.

Ben still felt the need to say, "Sorry I brought this up. I'm sure it's a source of great sadness for you. Maybe I can partially repay my debt to you for your love if I can listen when you feel down."

Their eyes met with a discovered new bond.

After Abraham left, Ben remembered, again with bright clarity, the day they first met, at the downtown Boston bus station.

"I think that's him!" Ben had cried, spying a tall, slender figure in a dark suit and fedora hat, a distinctly unusual looking man in the crowd as people filed out of the bus station.

"I think you're right!" Jacob said as he found a place to park. "I'll hop out and get him. Stay here in the car."

Not knowing what was expected of him, Jacob embraced his estranged brother warmly. Tears slid down Abraham's face as he returned the hug. Jacob wondered what Abraham must have endured over the past few weeks and months. Maybe he would talk about his experiences as he and his brother reacquainted themselves with one another. It was hard to know how it would go considering their years-long estrangement.

"Come, please follow me. Ben is in the car and can't wait to meet you."

"Thank you," he stammered, continuing to weep. "You have no idea how happy I am to see you and to feel safe after such a long time."

Abraham slid into the front passenger seat, turned around to look at Ben.

"This is Ben," Jacob said. "Meet your Uncle Abraham."

Ben offered his hand, believing this was the proper manly thing to do. Abraham took it gladly, kissing his nephew's hand and said in a deep baritone, "So glad to meet you, Ben."

"Sophie's home cooking one of her wonderful meals for us. Any foods you don't eat?" Jacob asked.

"I don't turn any food down, no matter what it is. I've given up that I must have kosher food. I'm grateful for any food."

Ben was leaning over the front seat to hear everything that was said, sizing up his uncle. He didn't have a beard, and his hair was not long, as his father had described. He had a faint odor of cigarettes. His complexion was sallow, with sunken cheeks. He reminded Ben of the statue of Lincoln at school. This Abraham was tall, like Lincoln, and there was a sadness about him, also like Lincoln. Ben liked his uncle already and imagined he had many stories to tell.

Jacob struggled to converse with his brother. They hadn't seen one another for over twenty years and their communication, never robust, had withered to a point that they were practically total strangers. Jacob didn't know how to break through this invisible barrier. Maybe, he thought, Ben could be his bridge.

"Ben, have any questions you want to ask Uncle Abraham?" Jacob said. Ben thought a minute and then said, "What was Canada like?"

"I was only there about a week," Abraham said in a subdued voice. "In Montreal. It reminded me a little of Europe. Old Europe, before the Nazis rose to power. But I didn't see much of the city. My French isn't good enough to ask how to get places, and I didn't know where I wanted to go anyway, so I stayed in my room most of the time."

"What did you do, all that time?" Jacob asked.

"There was a little library in the hotel lobby. I found a couple of books to read. My English is good. Also, newspapers. I love having newspapers once more. They were scarce in Hamburg before I left. Hitler saw to it that newspapers wouldn't let people know what was really happening. There's more news from Germany in Canada than I had in Hamburg. It shows how low my country has fallen."

Jacob finally said what had been on his mind since he'd gotten his brother's letter. "I wondered how you managed to get out of Germany. We heard there were no ways Jews could escape."

"I really don't want to talk about any of that," Abraham said with finality.

Jacob had read about "shell shock" that happened to many soldiers in the World War. Most people suffering from the collection of symptoms called "shell shock" refused to talk about their experiences during that grisly war, bottling up their horrific images of suffering and death. They often had nightmares, waking up in terror as their sleep-induced state allowed those buried memories to surface. Jacob wondered if Abraham might be suffering from this, even though he hadn't been in a conventional war. Jacob had read that emotional trauma—witnessing the horrors of war, watching what was happening to ordinary citizens subjected to the brutality of Nazi subjugation -- these could cause the equivalent of shell shock in non-combatants.

Ben broke up the drifting solemnity of the conversation. "Mother says you'll live in the spare bedroom at our house." Then, skipping to a completely different subject he asked, "Do you like dogs?"

"Not too much, Ben. The Nazis had a lot of big Shepherds they used to keep us in line. Those dogs had been trained to be vicious. Very scary."

"We have a really nice dog. His name is Slocum. I hope you and he can be friends," Ben said. "He's never bitten anybody. He likes to be petted and runs to fetch balls in our backyard. We have a big backyard, and I throw the ball, and he brings it back to me and then I throw it again. We have a lot of fun," Ben said, letting the words flow freely now that he had a chance to talk to his uncle. He rambled on, "I have a lot of toys. Do you play chess? Maybe we can play chess together. You can probably beat me, but I'm pretty good at it. I can play checkers too. Do you play checkers?"

Abraham chuckled at Ben's garrulousness. He could see he would be a great source of amusement and happiness in his new surroundings. He was reminded of his young patients in Hamburg. He always had enjoyed the children -- they cheered him up with their smiles and playfulness. They used to pull on his beard when he had one. Abraham would poke them gently in their tummies and make a squeaking sound, sure to arouse a big giggle.

Jacob pulled into his garage, honking his horn to alert Sophie. Ben was out of the car first, ran to open the door to Abraham, who smiled broadly for the first time in a long while. The warmth of this family was washing over him, and his melancholy began to lift.

"I'll take you right away to your room, show you the bathroom where you can freshen up," Jacob said. "When you're ready, come on down to the living room and meet Sophie. I'll show you around the house after we have dinner."

"Thank you for your kindness, Jacob. I'm so grateful. I haven't been so happy in months, maybe years. You and Ben have already given me hope."

"Oh, here's Sophie now. I guess I can show you to your room later."

"Welcome to America and our home," Sophie said with a warm smile. She opened her arms to Abraham, who awkwardly embraced her. Her light perfume was intoxicating. Abraham nearly fainted with the overwhelming emotions he felt.

"Thank you, thank you," he said, and once more, tears began to flow. "I should have brought you something, but I had nowhere to buy anything," he said, clearly embarrassed at his oversight.

"Don't give it a thought. After your ordeal, that's the last thing I expected," Sophie said.

"Do you need anything before we sit down for dinner?" Jacob asked.

"I'm fine," Abraham said quietly.

"Here, sit down and let me serve all of you dinner," Sophie said as she brought in a steaming pot.

Once they were eating, conversation became easier. Especially Ben, who couldn't stop talking.

"I'll show you my school on Monday. Can you come on Monday? Maybe I can introduce you to my class during 'show and tell.' They'd love to hear about Germany and your trip."

"Slow down, Benji," Sophie interjected. "Poor Uncle Abraham just got here. You're rushing him too much. You need to ask your teachers first, and you ought to ask your uncle if he wants to do that at all. Give him a little time to get used to being here."

Abraham was staring into his plate, still self-conscious in his new "home," overwhelmed by the loving reception of his brother's family. "I'm not sure I'm ready to do all that," Abraham said. "Give me a little time. I need to know all of you before I start meeting other people. Is that alright with you?"

"Of course it is, Abraham. We'll take our time and let you tell us when and if you're ready," Sophie said, reaching out to touch his hand. Dear Sophie, thought Jacob, always reading the emotional state of everyone around her.

As Ben returned to the here and now, he was acutely aware of how fortunate he was to have Uncle Abraham in his life.

Chapter 6

Old Sayings

The pressure from his bladder awakened Ben early. He buzzed for the nurse.

"Good morning, Ben. What's up?"

"An urgent call of nature. I'd like to try the urinal again."

"I'll bring one right away."

She handed him the urinal, gave him an encouraging nod, and scooted out of the room. He took a deep breath, closed his eyes, focusing on relaxing his sphincter. After a few seconds he heard a trickle pinging against the side of the urinal. *Relief at last!* He continued the release for what seemed like a long time, a smile spreading across his face. *There's nothing so under-rated as being able to pee,* he mused.

He ate breakfast with a new sense of hope. He could hardly wait to tell Arlene, now not only his physical therapist but his confidante when she came to start his exercise regimen. Sophie, Jacob, and Abraham would all be encouraged with this piece of good news.

Would his uncle say, "See, I told you things would get better?" Did this mean his paralysis might go away too? That would be his first question he'd ask the entourage when they came to make rounds.

But Dr. Weller came by early without the rest of the care team, surprising Ben.

"I wanted to tell you about your spinal fluid, before rounds," he said. "The protein content was up and there are some white blood cells. These are consistent with polio, not absolutely diagnostic, but I think polio is the diagnosis. It's what we've all thought from the beginning, but now the lab work combined with your clinical picture is convincing." He looked directly at Ben. "I didn't want to tell you this in front of everyone. Wasn't sure what your reaction would be."

Ben took a few deep breaths before responding. Although he was pretty sure polio was what he had, hearing the confirmation from Dr. Weller felt like a weight that might pull him under. He closed his eyes and wondered how his parents, especially Sophie, would receive this news. He was glad Dr. Weller had told him apart from the team, so the tears now coming wouldn't be seen by them.

"Not surprised," he said, trying to put on a show of strength, wiping away the dampness under his eyes. "You know, I've had time to get used to this diagnosis," he lied. "Of course, I'd hoped there would be another, more benign, explanation for my symptoms, but deep down, this was what I thought all along." He looked out the window for a moment. "Before you told me that crappy news, I was going to tell you about my good news from this morning."

"What's the good news?" Weller asked, perplexed.

"I could pee. If this continues, I won't have to be cathed anymore. And my bowels will probably also move. I count that as good news." After a pause, he looked directly at Dr Weller as he asked his most pressing question, "Do you think the legs might come back?"

"I don't know," Dr. Weller said. "Those are the hardest three words for a doctor to say, but they're true for this damnable disease. We're learning new things about it each day. We know physical therapy helps. There's no telling what lies ahead. So, we must stay optimistic." He looked at Ben, whose downturned mouth belied his stoic affect, and then at his watch and said, "Sorry to cut this short, but I should join the team for rounds now. If you need someone to talk to further, I can come back after rounds. I can also have our social worker stop by."

"Thanks. Probably a good idea to have the social worker stop by too. I do have some bad moments. I'd like someone to talk to when the dark moods come. Those moods remind me of what Winston Churchill called his 'black dog.' Even he had his moments. I also need advice about how my parents can deal with this. My mother is already quite upset. She and my dad may need someone to talk to as well."

"I understand. I'll ask our social worker to see you and ask her about meeting with your folks. Her name is Susan Goodall. She's a real help," Dr. Weller said as he left.

Ben watched the door swing shut after Dr. Weller and turned toward the window. Deep groaning sobs, rolled out of his chest, with tears to match his sense of grief. *Why? Why me? I've tried to be a good person every day of my life!* But he didn't have long to dwell in this land of self-pity, as the door soon opened and in came the white-coated morning rounds staff. He quickly dried his tears on the bedsheets, his back to the group as it moved like an amoeba to encircle his bed.

"Good morning, Ben," said Dan, the chief resident. "How're you feeling today?" he said, noticing the flush of his cheeks. "Dr. Weller told me he told you the results of your spinal fluid labs. Any questions?"

"Not much to ask about. Seems like that's almost a clincher." He paused, then said, "I told Dr. Weller what I think is my good news. Did he tell you?"

"No, he never tells us anything," Dan said with a smile. "Thinks we have to figure out everything ourselves."

"I could pee this morning," Ben said.

A quiet but emphatic "Yes!" came from the group, all smiles, indicating they, too, thought this was good news.

Ben grinned at their response, his mood lightening up.

"Since you're doing better clinically and we've finished the diagnostic workup, we're considering transferring you to the rehab floor. Your physical therapist can work more intensively with you there. And Dr. Weller told us Susan Goodall will be looking in on you sometime today," Dan said.

"What should I expect in the rehab ward?" Ben asked, a little apprehensive about this turn of events.

"The good news is that it's more open and you'll have others there to talk to."

"The bad news?"

"No bad news, unless having more PT is bad news," he smiled.

"How long will I be there?"

"Probably a couple of weeks. Once the PT folks assess your needs and your progress, you'll go home. With lots of planning about the home environment since your mobility needs will need to be considered."

Ben reflected on that last statement. Where would his bed be at home? What about all the stuff that makes him feel at home in his upstairs bedroom? The half-bathroom on the first floor didn't have a shower or a bathtub. How would he get up and down the stairs? His mind leapt from one logistic problem to another.

"When does this all happen?" he said.

"Probably tomorrow. As you know, inpatient beds are precious and with this polio epidemic we're tight on beds. So, I'd say sooner rather than later."

"Will you be making rounds on me or is there a new team?"

"New team. They're great. They'll be able to spend more time with you than we have."

"Well, thanks to all of you for the good care you've given me. I'll miss seeing all of you." The team all waved goodbye as they left.

Ben felt even more lonely. He'd gotten used to these faces and their kindness. Now he'd be meeting a whole new cast of characters. He remembered the old paradox "there's nothing constant in the world but change."

Old sayings reminded Ben of his uncle. Why hasn't Uncle Abraham been to see me lately? His parents hadn't mentioned anything, but try as he might, he couldn't dismiss the thought that Abraham might be sick himself. He always felt he had a sixth sense about such things.

Once more, as he pondered his special relationship with his uncle, his thoughts reached back to the early days getting to know him. He recalled the three of them -- Jacob, Abraham, and himself -- in the library that morning soon after Abraham's cough had been a concern. Ben had closed his eyes and pretended to be asleep, but he heard the whole conversation. He was forgotten by both Jacob and Abe.

"Good morning, Abraham."

"*Guten morgen*, Jacob. Oh, I mean good morning. Force of habit."

"How are you feeling, now that you've had a couple of nights of good sleep?"

"Pretty well, all things taken into account." Abraham paused. "I do have a cough I can't seem to rid myself of. It started on the boat and won't go away."

"I heard you coughing this morning. Any idea what it is? You're a doctor, after all."

Abraham smiled and said, "You know the old saying about a doctor who diagnoses his own ailments? *'Ein Doktor, der seine eigene Krankheit diagnostiziert, hat einen Esel als Arzt und einen Dummkopf als Patienten.'* (A doctor who diagnoses himself has an ass for a physician and a fool for a patient)," he chuckled.

"I'm not sure what it is, but I am worried."

"I took the liberty of calling our family doctor," Jacob said. "He can see you at ten this morning."

Abraham was silent for a moment, then said,

"That's very kind of you," doubt clouding his eyes. "But you must understand. I'm very hesitant about getting involved with doctors or hospitals. My passport is counterfeit, you recall. If your doctor discovers that I have a reportable infectious disease, I could be deported!"

He spoke, pacing back and forth, his face flushing with fear, reflecting an accumulation of anxiety he'd held in check for weeks. The worst thing that could happen to him now would be to be found out and deported. Where to? Back to Germany? Jailed in this country as an illegal alien?

"I'm only trying to help, Abraham. What if you have pneumonia -- or something worse, like TB -- causing your cough? Whatever it is, it should be diagnosed and treated. I trust Dr. Lane. If we explain your situation to him, he'll be discreet, I'm sure."

"I know you're trying to be helpful, but you have no idea what I've lived through in Germany. There you can't trust anyone unless you know them well, and even then, it's risky."

"This is America, Abraham. It's not Germany. I can't stand idly by and watch your health deteriorate. I think you need a doctor."

"Thank you for your concern, Jacob. I don't mean to appear ungrateful, but I am afraid." He fixed his gaze on Jacob. "I don't want to be seen by your doctor!"

"Abraham, listen to me for a minute." Jacob hesitated before continuing. "Both Sophie and I are extremely worried about your cough." He took a deep breath. "Frankly, I'm also worried about one of us catching something from you. I'm especially worried about Ben. He's got asthma, is very susceptible to germs. He gets sick easily. He's missed a lot of school this year. We just can't take a chance having him get sick."

Ambivalence seemed to grab Abraham all at once. But as reality replaced fear and the prospect of putting Ben in danger took hold in his mind, he relented. After a few moments of silence, he said, "Alright, Jacob. I'll see your doctor. But please, let him know of my status and the dangers I face if I'm found out."

"Thank you, Abraham. I'll reenforce to Dr. Lane the need for confidentiality. I know he'll help us."

Ben recalled the upshot of the visit had been the finding of pneumonia, not tuberculosis as Abraham himself had feared. Dr. Lane had prescribed sulfa, a new drug for bacterial pneumonia.

~~~

Ben snapped back to the present as the transport team came to take him to the Harley Rehabilitation Unit. Soon after he arrived there, Susan Goodall came to see him.

"Dr. Weller told me to stop by and get to know you. He filled me in on your medical condition. So, how're you feeling now that you're in Harley?"

"A little apprehensive saying goodbye to those folks taking care of me for weeks. Will you be seeing me here?"

"That's the plan. I'll come by as often as you'd like once I've talked to you a little bit and you fill me in on all that's happened to you."

"Would it be possible for you to talk also to my parents? They're pretty upset about my paralysis."

"Of course, I'll be happy to talk to them. But," getting right to the point, "how're you feeling?"

"Not good."
~~~

"Do me a favor. Jot down what you're feeling and thinking, and we can use those notes to start our discussion when I come back tomorrow. What's a good time for you?"

"After PT, I guess. Can you check with Arlene as to when she will be done torturing me?"

Susan smiled. "Sure, I'll do that. I like your sense of humor. That'll help in the long run. See you tomorrow!"

Chapter 7

Harley

The Harley Rehabilitation Center was an innovation at the Pediatric Hospital housed in a separate building. The main floor, where physical therapy took place, was a sprawling complex with the latest design in exercise equipment. The inpatient beds were in four-bed wards on a different floor. There was an emerging body of evidence that patients having social interactions as part of their healing process played a significant role in recovery.

On his first day in the exercise room, Ben was disoriented and bewildered by seeing so many people with serious physical impairments. He looked at his fellow patients with a mixture of curiosity and dread. *All these cripples*, he thought, having not yet come to grips that he was one of them. As he surveyed his new environment from his wheelchair, Pauline, his new physical therapist, walked in. "How do you like your new place?" she asked in an upbeat voice.

"Taking a while to get used to the idea if you want the truth. So many people with so many problems. It sort of confirms what I've been trying to deny-- that I'm disabled. So, if I seem a little lost, that's part of the reason."

"I understand how it can be a bit of a jolt as you look around. For someone whose life has been smooth sailing, the reality of this place can be tough. The patients you see are here for all kinds of reasons. Some were in injured in falls, or auto crashes, birth accidents, and some are here only to rehab from surgical procedures. They're from all age groups.

"I haven't known you very long, but I see in you a reservoir of strength to rise to this challenge. Once we get going on our program, I know you'll find your way towards acceptance.

"So, let me tell you what we hope to accomplish and how we'll approach it," she said. She sat down next to Ben and handed him a sheaf of papers describing the exercises he would be doing and explanations as to what they were intended to do.

"Want to begin?" she asked.

"Why not? That's why I'm here, I guess."

Pauline went easy on Ben for his first day. A short time after she was finished, Susan Goodall appeared. She was a full-figured woman of fifty-five and pleasant demeanor. She sat on a chair next to bed, and in a low and reassuring voice said, "Did you make a list?"

"A short one. But enough to get started, I think."

"What's first?"

"Will I be able to do my job as a doctor?"

"What area of medicine are you thinking about?"

"Haven't completely decided, but I think pediatrics."

"Any particular reason for that?"

"Well, I was happiest while on my pediatric rotation. Maybe because I identified with the kids, never having grown up myself." Ben laughed, a little embarrassed that he was sharing this idea with this woman he barely knew. "I think the other reason is that children, in their naivete, have so much hope, you can't help but get inspired by their optimism."

"Let's explore that a little more. Is there a particular role you see yourself playing in pediatrics?"

"One of my projects in high school was working in a daycare center. I enjoyed teaching little kids about science, fascinated by how fast they learned and understood things. I've always enjoyed teaching."

"How about teaching medical students?"

"I'd like that too. Yeah, I'm inspired by my mentors and can see myself doing that." He hesitated, then said, "That's a really good idea. Why didn't I think of that myself?"

"You probably did, but the thought passed.

"What do you see as barriers in, as you say, doing your job as a doctor?"

"Isn't that obvious?"

"I want to know what you see as barriers, not the fact of your paralysis," Susan said in a lowered voice, recognizing Ben's sensitivity.

"I don't see how someone who can't walk can take care of patients. That's a real barrier, as I think about it."

"I could see not walking or standing a problem if you wanted to be a surgeon," Susan said. "But it doesn't prevent your seeing patients. Or teaching. Or advising students. Or running a clinic. Or doing research. Or writing. Lots of things you can do. And I think that's the main point I would make today. Emphasize the things you can do and then do them."

"One thing I should be doing," Ben said. "Studying. I'm missing the intellectual stimulation of being in a learning environment."

"Do you have medical books at home?"

"Oh yeah, they assigned thick books on internal medicine, pediatrics, surgery, etcetera. They're at home gathering dust."

"Any reason you couldn't read them here?" Susan asked.

"None. Why didn't I think of that?" Ben said. "I'll ask Mother to bring them here. I have plenty of time to study them and it would make the time pass quicker. I guess I could also ask a couple of classmates to lend me their lecture notes. Stay up to date that way. What a great idea! Thanks!"

"Okay, next time I come you can fill me in on the latest advances in medicine," she said with a twinkle in her eyes.

Ben regarded Susan intently as she spoke, and his mind raced as he rolled all these possibilities around in his mind. Good advice, he thought. I see why Dr. Weller sent her to me. I need to hear more from this woman.

~~~

After Susan left, a knock on the door.

"Come in," Ben said

Two of his classmates, Stan O'Brien and David Littlefield strolled in.

"How're you doin' these days?" Stan said.

"Taking each day as it comes," Ben said. "Today's a pretty good day. Just finished talking with Susan Goodall, a social worker Dr. Weller suggested. Good advice from her."

"Well, we're sort of representatives of the class. Everyone's thinking about you and wondering how you're making out. Got this card for you," David said, handing Ben a get-well card with signatures all over it.

"Well, thanks! I've been thinking about you guys too. What service are you on now?"

"I'm on surgery, he's on Ear, Nose and Throat," Stan said. "I'm really interested in ortho, so I like this rotation a lot."

"I'm going to be on the cancer ward next week. Doubt I'll go into that, but I am interested in Hematology. We'll see," David said. "Do you have any idea when you'll be coming back?"
~~~

"Remains to be seen. A lot of bridges to cross before that. I don't even know whether they'll let me return."

"That's a lot of bull hockey," Stan said. "Of course, they'll let you back. We'll go on strike if they give you a hard time."

"Well, I've fallen behind pretty much. That reminds me-- any way you could get lecture notes that I missed? That would really be helpful, and it would occupy my mind, so it doesn't atrophy."

"That's no problem," O'Brien said. "I'll collect them from the best note-takers in the class -- the girls -- who also have the best handwriting. I'll bring them by. How long will you be here?"

"Not sure, but I guess at least a couple of more weeks," Ben said. "Thank everyone for the card. And thanks ahead of time for the lecture notes."

After they left, Ben's mind was crowded with thoughts about how many people were helping him get through this and how he was so fortunate to have the family and friends that he had. Self-pity was a luxury he couldn't afford.

Over the next two weeks, Sophie and Jacob visited him daily. They brought him the books he'd asked for. Often Sophie stayed after Jacob left, to watch him being put through the paces of physical therapy. She wanted to learn everything possible about his exercises so she could be sure Ben did them correctly at home.

Susan Goodall met with Sophie and Jacob one of the days they came to see Ben. He was not present during their session because Susan, with wisdom gained from experience, asked him to understand it was to be therapy session with his parents and his presence would have made the dynamic much different. He was curious as to what transpired, so he asked Sophie.

"Well, Susan was wonderful. We're going to meet with her regularly for talks after you come home. She explained many things we wondered about and gave us good advice about our feelings, things we haven't discussed with anyone. As I said, she was great.

"We're excited about what we're doing at home. We're putting in a new bathroom in the downstairs lav," Sophie said. "It's going well and will be ready when you come home. Can't wait to have you home where you belong. I've also been talking to Pauline and she's giving me tips on things we'll need so you can get around your new 'apartment.'

"You look like you've lost weight. Are you eating enough?" Sophie asked, concern creasing her forehead.

"Appetite's picking up. I'll be glad to have your cooking though. Hospital food is notoriously awful." He hesitated asking Sophie the question that had been worrying him for a couple of weeks. After he got his courage up, he said,

"Is Uncle Abraham sick or something? He hasn't been in to see me in a while."

"Um, well, yes, he has been sick. We haven't seen him for a while either, so I called him yesterday. He's had some abdominal pain and intestinal problems. He's seeing his doctor today. Perhaps we'll know more after that. I'll let you know."

"How old is he now?" Ben asked.

"Late sixties, I think. He's ten years older than your father who's fifty-eight, but Abe has been in good health after those first days with us when he had that cough. Remember? Dr. Lane got him through that with my help and good food!"

"Yeah, I remember that cough and how worried you were. When you talk to him tell him I miss him and when I get home, I hope he can come see me." *If this were six weeks ago, I'd be going to see him. Another change in my life.*

~~~

When the day came for Ben to go home, he felt wildly ambivalent.

After several weeks in the rehab unit, he'd been absorbed into a group of people who were more caring and helpful than any group of human beings he'd ever known. They'd become like family, even more familiar and intimate than his real family. They'd seen every inch of his body, held his hand through difficult times, reassured him repeatedly, and demonstrated they cared about him, much like his own parents and uncle
~~~

did. He knew the minutiae of his hospital milieu by virtue of his total immersion in it.

He would, at least for a while, miss this community—the smells, noises, and yes, even the bad food. But he was eager to go home, learn about navigating his now circumscribed world with his altered body and new expectations.

Once his possessions were thrust into two paper shopping bags, along with his books, post discharge instructions and a plethora of follow-up appointments, he was helped into a wheelchair and rolled out to the nursing station, with Jacob and Sophie lugging the shopping bags. Ben soon learned that crutches, canes, a walker, and various home health aides -- urinals, shoehorns, devices to help get stockings on -- had already been delivered to their home the day before.

He was startled to see the nursing and house staff, attending physicians, social workers, therapists, housekeepers, and transportation workers all assembled around the nursing station, with balloons and posters wishing him well. A cheer went up and "for he's a jolly good fellow" sung in unharmonious unison. Choral singing was not the forte of the hospital staff. A box of greeting cards, some funny, some achingly sincere, was handed to him.

"Whoa, turn this wheelchair around, I want to stay!" he laughed, and then tears came as people shook his hands, kissing the top of his head, pressing little gifts into his hand as he passed. Sophie broke into tears and even Jacob struggled to keep his composure they were so moved by this outpouring of affection for their son. It was obvious they felt he was a special person, and it took twenty minutes to navigate the wheelchair to the exit of the Harley Rehab Center for all the well-wishing.

Getting into the car was a new experience. Louis, the transportation guy, dwarfing everyone else, was most helpful lifting Ben bodily, his flaccid legs dangling, out of the wheelchair and carefully depositing him in the back seat of their sedan.

"Can we take you home with us?" Jacob said to Louis, with a smile of gratitude and an offer of a tip, which Louis graciously declined. Ben, as he struggled to position himself in his seat, wondered if the family would have to get a different kind of car with more room, perhaps a station wagon, to cart him places. He also wondered how, as Jacob intimated when he kidded Louis about coming home with them, they would manage to get him out of the car and into the house. His father was not strong enough to lift him the way Louis did, and Ben realized once more this was the beginning of a steep learning curve of adjustment.

When they pulled into the driveway Ben saw that his parents had arranged for help getting him out of the car and into the house. Two young men carefully maneuvered him out of his seat and into a wheelchair, then into the house on a new ramp from the driveway to the kitchen door.

Ben marveled at the transformation. In his new first floor bedroom stood a hospital bed with frames attached overhead containing several fixtures that he would use to position himself for getting out of bed and into a walker or onto crutches when the time came for that. Under the window was a comfortable-looking loveseat with an attached tray for reading or meals. The bathroom, with raised toilet seat, was decorated in sparkling white tile walls. The shower was equipped with a built-in seat and rails at waist level. All around the rooms were rails for gripping. Sophie and Jacob had thought of everything.

As he took it all in, Sophie and Jacob stood at the door waiting to see his response.

"This is fantastic! You're the best parents in the world!" Ben said, with a mixture of gratitude and regret that this all had to be done for him. Sophie rushed to his side, knelt at the side of the wheelchair, and gave him an awkward hug. "We hope we've thought of everything you'd need, but please, Ben, tell us what else you need as you start living here." Jacob stood next to him, resting his hand on Ben's shoulder. Tears gathered in all their eyes.

"So, what would you like to eat?" Sophie said, breaking the mood, eager to begin her now role as chief caretaker.

"What's available?" Ben said, knowing Sophie had been obsessive about her shopping for his first meal at home.

"Soups, salads, sandwiches, drinks--the whole shebang."

"Why don't you just make what you think I'd like, Mom. I'll enjoy it, whatever you make."

After lunch they all rested in his new room, he in his wheelchair and Sophie and Jacob on the loveseat. Sophie beamed as she looked at Ben, glad to have her boy back home. Jacob sat quietly, but his face reflected his relief that his only child was at home, albeit under utterly new and different circumstances. He'd planned the remodeling with his jeweler's precision and was pleased that it was to Ben's liking. They made small talk for a time, then Ben asked, "What about Uncle Abraham?"

Sophie turned to Jacob. "Can you tell him?"

Jacob pulled himself up out of his comfortable slouch in the loveseat.

"Well. I guess the only way to say this is to call it like it is. He has cancer," Jacob said slowly. "That's why he hasn't been to see you. He didn't want us to tell you until you got home so it wouldn't hinder your recuperation. But he gave us permission to tell you once you were home."

What else can I bear? I was worried that something like that was going on.

But rather than revealing his own anguish, he switched to his professional demeanor and said, "Where's the cancer?"

"Pancreas. But the doctors told us it's already spread." Jacob said.

"Is he feeling awfully sick?"

"Yes, unfortunately. He's lost about twenty pounds, has little appetite and very low energy."

"Can he get around at all? He's not in the hospital?"

"No, he's at home in his apartment, has an all-day nurse, Lila, who's a peach. She prepares three meals each day, including supper before she leaves. But he can't move around very well."

"Can I go see him?"

"We can take you to see him. He'd like that. Maybe tomorrow?"

"Can we go today?" He knew the prognosis for pancreatic cancer was miserable.

"Do you really feel up to it? You just got home. You must be very tired," Sophie said.

"Hold on, you two. We're getting the new car tomorrow," Jacob said. "It's a 1952 Chevrolet Suburban and it's huge! We're to pick it up in the morning. We'll have to wait 'til then to see Abraham."

Though disappointed, Ben saw the logic of this. But his concern for his uncle carried him on the tide back to when Abraham first came to live with them and had an illness that had caused all of them to worry.

Chapter 8

Recollections, 1939

"Benjie, good news!" Mother said, "Abraham got a good report from Dr. Lane. We're going to have a festive dinner tonight. And you can have time with your uncle again!"

"Yay, yay! Is he around right now?" I said, coming in from school, tossing my fourth-grade books on the side table.

"He's in the library, I think. He was calling his friend at MIT about a job there," she said. "He may still be there but go in quietly if he's still on the phone."

I grabbed an apple from the bowl on the table and ran to the library. I saw Abraham pacing around the room, a broad smile on his face.

"Hi Uncle Abraham!" I really startled him.

"Hi Ben. You gave me a fright! So good to see you! Come, sit down. Tell me about your day. And then I'll tell you my good news."

"We're studying mosquitoes," I said. "Didya know only bites from female mosquitoes cause malaria?" I'd failed to pick up on his excitement about his conversation with his friend at MIT in my typical ten-year-old self-centeredness.

"Well, Ja, I did know that. I'm a doctor, remember?"

"Well, even doctors don't know everything," I said, smiling at Uncle Abraham. "Did you ever see malaria?"

"Not in Germany. I did see some cases when I was in Africa."

"Really, you were in Africa?" I said, looking with renewed admiration at my uncle.

"An elective during medical school. An elective allows you to choose what to study and where, for one whole month. I chose Kenya, in Africa."

"Why there?"

"Different culture, one I knew nothing about. Different maladies--diseases--there, and they live in ways unfamiliar to me. I wanted to see and experience how they live."

As I considered what I was hearing from Abraham, he became more and more fascinating to me. *What would it be like to be him? To live in Africa. Even to live in Germany.*

"I'm thinking about being a doctor. But I dunno. Seems like an awful lotta work," I said, trying to elicit a response from Abraham.

"Being a doctor does take a lot of effort, but I never thought of it as work. I love studying diseases, how they come about, what causes them, how to diagnose and treat them. It keeps the mind churning all the time."

"Do you have to be real smart?"

"The main thing you need is desire and curiosity. The other thing you need is a sense of duty. A sense of community, like we're all in this together."

"What are those things? I don't understand what you're talkin' about," I said.

"Being a practicing doctor is a calling. It's not just a job or a way to make a living. It's a sense that you must do this. Sort of a religious experience. You just know."

"Hmm. I don't get it. Who calls you?"

"That's a good question, the answer to which I do not have. It's that voice in your head that tells you what's right and wrong, what you should do. I don't know where it comes from. Some people believe it's from God, others believe it's from your family or community or something else.

"Let me give you an example. One day, as I was finishing seeing patients and extremely tired, I sat down in my office with a cup of tea. A repeated knocking at the door alarmed me. I opened it to see a woman, weeping and agitated, walking around in circles outside the door. I asked her what was wrong, what was upsetting her.

"She told me her eight-year-old little girl was having one of her fits and she had done everything she knew but couldn't stop her from shaking. "Take me to her right away," I told her. We hurried to where she lived, down a dark alley and into a dank cellar. This little tyke was lying on the dirty floor, still foaming at the mouth, her arms and legs quivering, her eyes rolled back in her head."

"I picked her up, cradled her in my arms, and ran back with her to the office, her mother close behind me. In my office, I gave her an injection of a calming medicine and waited. It didn't do much, so I gathered her up again and went to my car, her mother jumping in the back seat, and we drove quickly to the hospital. The doctors and nurses there flew into action, giving her oxygen and, after asking me what I'd already given her, gave her another shot to stop the shaking. After a few minutes she finally stopped shaking. Her mother broke down in sobs, hugged me and I must admit I was overcome with relief and shed a few tears as well.

"After this was over, I was exhausted, both from the long day I'd had in the office, but also from the emotional strain of this poor child's ordeal. But I also felt content. I'd done something important for that family.

"That satisfaction is what I get from being a doctor. That's why I say it is a calling."

"Hmm. I guess I have to think about that some more," I said.

"Keep trying to figure it out," Abraham said, smiling at Ben. "It'll only take you a lifetime."

"I used to think that grownups knew the answers to all kinds of questions. But I see Mother and Dad not knowing about a lot of things."

"Any grownup who tells you they have all the answers, you should not listen to them." He paused, thinking. "There's an old saying: He who knows not, and knows not that he knows not, is a fool. Don't believe him."

"Sometimes I don't understand everything you say. Like that old saying you just told me."

"I can write it down for you and you can study it."

"Another thing I'd like to know, Uncle. How'd you get out of Germany?"

"Where shall I start?" Abraham began. "I guess you would be interested to know how I got out of my city—Hamburg—first. Shall I begin there?"

"Yeah."

"I made many friends in our poor community. Everyone knew me and I think most liked me. I had a couple of enemies, of course, patients who didn't get well and blamed me. But mostly, people took care of each other.

"Two of my patients were men who worked on the wharves along the Elbe River. That river becomes very wide as it enters the bay and there is much commerce taking place on the river. I made friends with these two men because I had learned they were helping Jews escape Hamburg by hiding in ship's holds.

"One day, when one of them was in my office, I expressed the fear we all had about what was happening in our country.

"'Do you want to get out before it is too late? I can arrange it,' he said."

"I wanted to say goodbye to all my patients, but that would have been dangerous. There was no telling who might be in league with the SS."

"What's the SS?" I asked.

"That was short for Schutzstaffel, the terrible police unit that did so many bad things to Jews. I had gotten several threatening calls from the SS that I should watch my step. I am certain those threats would have been carried out soon. I felt terrible about my decision, but I knew I had to leave.

"One thing led to another, and I soon found myself headed to the port with the man who had arranged everything. As we approached the ship I was to board, we saw two SS officers making their rounds. We circled around, shipyard sounds dampening our movements, and finally I joined the crowd getting aboard, hoping we had not been detected. It was very frightening. I soon found myself in the hold of a freight vessels bound for Canada. A few other refugees and I had managed to avoid capture and certain execution. We felt reasonably safe where wee were.

"It took a long time to get across the ocean and I was sick most of the way, you know, seasick. There were several others just as sick as I was, all miserable. But we had hope.

"I felt sad and guilty, leaving my patients, but things were getting worse by the day. I had been threatened by the Nazis at the pharmacy frequently because I annoyed them, asking for more medicines for my patients. One of them told me these dirty people didn't deserve any help and that if I kept complaining they would stop all supplies.

"Under these circumstances there was little I could do. So, I decided to survive. I still feel terrible about deserting my patients and probably will always feel that way. I lose sleep over it. But what is done is done."

"They could've arrested you or even killed you if you stayed, dad says. Sounds like you were an annoyance. That's what mother calls me sometimes."

"Yes, I was definitely an annoyance."

"When you got to Canada, how did you get off the boat and not get caught?"

"There was a small group in Montreal, French-speaking men with relatives in the French Resistance who were part of this business of smuggling refugees. The Quebec government looked the other way since it was such a small operation. These men prepared fake papers for us, so we slipped into the country with no notice by immigration agents. Or perhaps they just turned a blind eye to what was going on. You want to know my new name?"

"You're not Abraham?"

"No. I am now Eric Werner. My new fake passport has this name on it. They told me to shave my beard and cut my hair and they took a picture of me for my passport."

"Did you have any money?"

"I took all the money I had in my office. Not a lot, but enough to get by for a few weeks," Abraham (now Eric Werner) said. "That's where Bernard Weiner, my friend at the Massachusetts Institute of Technology, gave me so much help. He even gave me a job at MIT. I've been very lucky."

Chapter 9

Visit to Cambridge, 1953

The ride in their new car to see Uncle Abraham was shrouded in silence. Sophie and Jacob were hesitant to say much about his condition to Ben, who stared blankly at the Charles River as they passed over the Longfellow Bridge into Cambridge. His forehead was wrinkled not only from the glare of the sun, but from the strain of worry. He knew from his studies that pancreatic cancer had a grim prognosis, almost a sure death sentence. He was beginning his own grieving even before he saw him.

Swinging onto Memorial Drive, Jacob looked for Abraham's apartment, then was frustrated in a search for parking. He double-parked in front of the apartment building, unloaded Ben's wheelchair, helped him into his chair and then scurried back into the car to continue his quest for a parking space.

"This is so awkward," Ben muttered as he and Sophie waited on the sidewalk. "It's gonna take time getting used to working this damned wheelchair. Physical therapists don't tell you about everyday indignities of being disabled, like now, stranded on a sidewalk until your father can come and help you. Like being a two-year-old."

"I don't know what to say," Sophie fumbled out the words. "You know, you can still do a lot of things. You should thank God for that. You can scoff at my Pollyanna attitude, or even get mad at me for my optimism, but things, you know, will get better as you learn how to manage them." She looked around for Jacob to rescue her from this conversation. She patted Ben on his arm, the only thing she could think to do, as his grumbling subsided.

"I had to park in the public garage on Memorial, that's what took so long. Sorry," Jacob said on his return.

Arriving at Abraham's unit, they knocked and waited. When the door slowly opened, Ben was stunned by how much Abraham had aged since he last saw him: sunken cheeks, dark circles outlining his eyes, like a prize fighter's face after a match, his dark and wrinkled clothes hanging loosely on his frame.

He opened his arms to Ben, who reached his arms up from his wheelchair, tears rolling down his cheeks, wishing he could embrace Abraham properly. Another dispiriting token of his condition, added to a growing litany of regret.

"So glad you've come," Abraham whispered, his voice weakened and hoarse. "I'll get out of your way so you can move your chair in." Ben, getting more adept at using his wheelchair, maneuvered it into the living room, followed by Jacob and Sophie.

"Can I get you some tea or coffee?" Abraham asked.

"No thanks, we had breakfast not too long ago, so I'll pass," Ben said.

"Likewise, for us," Jacob said. "Thanks just the same."

"Ben, first tell me how you're doing," Abraham said, in his familiar manner of directing the subject of conversation to others.

"Slowly getting adjusted, Uncle Abe." He was unsure how to proceed. He wanted to know more about Abraham's situation but decided to allow that to spool out on its own. "This is all new to me, as you can imagine. But these two," nodding towards his parents, "have been great, helping, and getting the house ready. Does he know about the remodeling?" he turned, asking Sophie.

"We've told him all about it, but he's not seen it yet," she said, and addressing Abraham, "When can you come to see what we've done?"

"Well, you know, I'm quite unsteady on my feet, so I prefer staying here, close to my bathroom and other familiar things. But thanks for the offer, Sophie."

Seizing the opportunity to find out about his uncle, Ben asked, "How do you get along here by yourself?"

"Ah, I have a pleasant woman who comes each day to help me with meals and such. She offered to come more often but so far, I manage by myself. A nurse from the hospital comes after lunch to check my blood pressure and give me my pills. They tell me I'm doing well, so I guess it's so.

"But I want to know about you, Ben," he said, predictably, always thinking of others. "You say you're getting adjusted, that's Sehr gut." He paused, regarding Ben with his astute and knowing gaze, saying, "What are you most worried about?"

"I have a whole list," Ben said with an impish smile. "Let's see. I guess, first on the list, is how am I able to continue medical school and work on the hospital wards? What will patients think about a crippled doctor? Then after that, how am I gonna get places? From home to school and on hospital floors, things I used to take for granted. I can't drive, so I'll need a driver. Mom can't be available for all these trips."

"Au contraire, Benji. I'm available for whatever you need," Sophie interrupted. "I don't have much to do at home."

"I've been checking into that matter, Ben," Jacob offered. "Found out there are accessories in cars these days for people who can't use their legs. Takes some training to learn to drive using them, but it's one solution."

"Hmm, but what about getting in and out of the car, in and out of the wheelchair? Getting the wheelchair out of the car? These are problems too."

Abraham was silent listening to his nephew's angst. He would have sacrificed anything to have prevented Ben's paralysis. After spending a lifetime caring for patients with every kind of disease and confronting the travail only health workers see, one would assume he would have become inured to pathos. But now, when his beloved nephew is stricken, Jacob and Sophie could see that his pain was as intense as that he'd described, like the first time he faced a patient with a dreadful condition. For all three of them, thoughts of other problems in their lives fell away as they contemplated the cruel turn Ben's life had taken.

"I'm not going to give you empty platitudes about your misfortune," Abraham said in a near whisper. "You've been handed some bad luck. But you can't allow it to embitter you, or you will have lost twice.

"You mentioned love the last time we spoke. I think you were talking then about romantic love between two people. That is naturally on your list. But remember, love comes in many forms: romantic love, love of a mother for her children, brotherly love, love of your country, your community. For me, I found early in life that love of my work, treating the sick, meant so much to me. Giving oneself over to something bigger than yourself is most fulfilling. Remember one time I talked about medicine being a calling?"

"I was just thinking about that the other day," Ben said. "I've never forgotten it."

Jacob looked at Sophie as tears came to his eyes. Having his brother here had turned out to be such a blessing for their family.

"I'm now very tired so I have to lie down," Abraham said. "I'm so glad you've come to see me. I hope you'll come again. But soon. One never knows."

As they left, Jacob lingered behind.

"Abe, I wanted to thank you for all you've done for Ben, and for us as a family. I don't know what stroke of fate sent you to us, but it's been a blessing to have you among us for these past few years. I just can't thank you enough."

"It is I who should be thanking you, Jacob. Without your kindness in taking me in I would have been desperate." After all the years of disaffection, the brothers embraced. Both sensed it would be for the last time.

On the way back to Brookline, they all were filled with mixed feelings of closeness with Abraham and sober comprehension of how short his remaining time was amongst them. On the ride home, not a word was spoken.

Chapter 10

The Letters

To: Stanley Stevens, M.D., Dean
Channing Medical School
100 Longmeadow Avenue
Boston, MA 02116

Dear Dr. Stevens,

I am a third-year medical student at Channing Medical School. As you may be aware, I contracted poliomyelitis during this past summer while on my rotation in pediatrics. Due to a resulting paralysis below the waist, I must rely on a wheelchair for mobility.

I am eager to continue my studies and graduate, if possible, with my class. I have no doubt I will prevail over my disability and look forward to a long career in medicine. I am writing for advice about the resumption of my medical school education.

Please let me know how I should proceed.
Sincerely,
Ben Levinson, third-year Channing Medical School student

~~~

As he finished writing, he scanned his room. His parents had done a spectacular job in fitting out his living space, providing every possible aid to his mobility. He had gradually learned to move from his state-of-the-art hospital bed to wheelchair, to bathroom, to shower and toilet, and was already bathing himself, saving the embarrassment of having anyone else help him with this private endeavor.

Two triangular bars attached to the ceiling, one above his bed and one adjacent to the bed, served as transfer stabilizers as he moved from a supine position in bed to his wheelchair. One of his wheelchairs was waterproof, suitable for use in what he called his 'drive-in' shower stall, and another was for general use. Jacob had gotten a set of parallel bars for Ben to do physical therapy, hoping some function would return in his legs. The bars also helped develop his upper body strength, critical as he moved from one position to another.

With the letter to the dean, Ben hoped to take charge of his immediate future. If Uncle Abraham was right, there should be a clear path to resume his education. But until he got confirmation, he couldn't be sure. What puzzled him was that no one from the medical school had contacted him since he'd become ill. He'd also had heard nothing from Dr. Weller or Dr. Woolhandler, both of whom knew his case from the
~~~

beginning. He wondered if he should try to get in touch with either of them. *Why not?*

"Hello, this is Ben Levinson, a third-year medical student. I'm trying to reach Dr. Weller at the Student Health Service at Boston Pediatric Hospital. Can you either connect me to his office or give me a number I can call?"

"I'll try to connect you, sir. If you don't reach his office, his direct number is 617-555-1212. Stay on the line."

Ben took a deep breath and waited. There was the sound of ringing, over ten signals. He held on for a few more, but then he tried dialing the direct number.

"Dr. Weller's office. Ellie speaking. Who's calling?"

"Oh, hello, Ellie. Good to hear your voice. This is Ben Levinson. Remember me?"

"Ben, how could I forget you? One of our favorite patients! How are you, for heaven's sake? We knew you'd been in Harley, but the press of other cases kept us occupied. We should have been in touch. Sorry."

"Understood, Ellie. Well, the good news is that I'm home now. The not-so-good news is that I'm paralyzed from the waist down."

"Yes. We did know that since you were in Harley." An awkward pause. "I'm so sorry." Ben could hear it in her voice. He couldn't help but wonder why they hadn't called or at least sent a card. But he let it go. That was history.

"I'm so glad you called so we can reconnect. Did you want to talk to Dr. Weller?"

"Well, um, yes. I need to ask him some questions. Is he available?"

"Not now, but he should be back in a couple of hours. Can I have him call you?"

"Yes, please." He gave her his number, and after a few pleasantries, ended the call.

Am I so self-centered that I suppose everyone in the world is waiting to hear of my recovery? Maybe I can talk to Susan Goodall about my feelings of being ignored. Don't they understand how hard this is for a normal, vigorous young stud like me to accept that I'm only half a man now? What girl wants a cripple for a mate? Can I even reproduce if any gal would have me? I can't even play a game of touch football. I can't ever again dive off the high board. No marathons for me.

Stop it! I need to focus on those things that have been done for me instead of whining that the cruel world doesn't care about me, woe is me, wallowing in self-pity. I'm surrounded by the love of my family. Not everyone -- in fact, very few people -- enjoy the advantages I've always had. Loving parents, a home in an affluent suburb of a major city, a great education. Most importantly, an opportunity to make a difference in the world.

As the rhythm of his mind skipped from one thought to another, it was interrupted by the phone. He picked up the receiver.

"Ben, is that you?" Weller said.

"Yes. Dr. Weller?"

"Yeah, good to hear your voice. How're you doing? You home?"

"Yes, home, with my family. And so glad to be here."

"I've been following your progress through my spies. So, I know your medical status. What I don't know is how you're reacting to it. Tell me something about your state of mind."

"I have mostly discouraging days if you want the truth. I'm trying to 'accept those things I cannot change' as the saying goes, but it's hard. You know, when things have always gone wonderfully well all your life, you kinda' expect that to always be the case. Must be part of youth. The lack of experience in confronting bad turns of luck. Sorta spoiled, to be honest."

"I understand. I think your analysis is pretty on-target. Do you have any questions that have gone unanswered by all the people taking care of you?"

"My main worry now is, will the medical school allow me to continue?"

"I'm unable to speak for the medical school, but my opinion is not to worry. I can't imagine there would be any question you'd be encouraged to continue. I'll put in my two cents to the dean's office for whatever that's worth. I'm only a health center doctor, not a faculty don."

"Thanks, Dr. Weller. I'll be grateful for your help."

When the conversation ended, Ben felt a little better. But he'd feel more encouraged once he got a reassuring answer from the dean's office. His uncle was right. Giving yourself over to something bigger than yourself is a driving force of life. Something that keeps you going.

Ben had to wait several days for a response from the dean's office. When it came, he tore it open expectantly.

Dear Mr. Levinson,
Your letter has been received. I've forwarded it to Mr. Garvey, Assistant Dean for Student Affairs. He will respond to your inquiry.
Sincerely,
Stanley Stevens, MD
Dean, Channing Medical School.

"Well, shit!" Ben shouted when he read the letter. "What a lame response that is! No indication of what the decision might be. I've been turned over to some administrator who never went to medical school, has no knowledge of what it takes to study medicine. What kind of crap is this?" he said to the walls of his bedroom, feeling now like this was a prison.

He wanted to pick up the phone and call the dean and scream into his ears. But as he got over his anger, his cooler head knew he wouldn't be allowed to speak directly to the dean and anyway, that kind of behavior would get him nowhere fast.

But he didn't have to wait long. Two days later, he received a letter from Garvey.

Dear Mr. Levinson,

Dr. Stevens sent your letter to me. I've discussed this with three members of the Committee. They are asking for you to come and meet with them. Call my office at your earliest convenience to set up a time to meet.

Our office is in the main medical school on Longmeadow Avenue.
Sincerely,

William Garvey, Assistant Dean, Student Affairs, Channing Medical School

Ben read the letter once, then twice and a third time. He couldn't believe it. He was already a third-year medical student. He'd had excellent grades for the first two years, in the upper ten percent of the class, and now they're asking him to meet with some Committee.

Calm down. Take a deep breath.

He called and set up a date for the following week. His face was flushed, his heart beating wildly. He knew his blood pressure was up; he could feel it pulsating in his ears.

He didn't know which way to turn. With his anxiety level hitting the ceiling, he called Dr. Weller's office. Ellie answered.

"Hi Ben, how're you doing?" she said, the ever-present smile in her voice.

"Well, not good," Ben said. He told her the problem and asked for Dr. Weller to call.

"I'll tell him right away. You don't need this. I'm sorry they're putting you through this. It's not right."

"Thanks Ellie. It's all I can do to remain calm."

How he was going to tell his parents about this was the next hurdle. He had to collect himself and present an unperturbed front for his parents. His mother might go through the roof with anxiety, his father might get his umbrage up and call and threaten the medical school with a lawsuit. Who knows what could happen if everyone got upset? So, he had to maintain a placid front, even if he felt like his own Vesuvian eruption was imminent.

Chapter 11

The Committee

"I have an appointment next week to talk to a medical school committee about continuing," Ben told Jacob and Sophie at dinner. "I can't wait to see them," he lied. He couldn't shake his self-doubts, his overarching anxiety about his incapacities.

"Who will you be seeing?" Jacob asked.

"Um, there'll be three people."

"Meeting with a committee? You're not applying to medical school, you're already in your third year!" Jacob exploded, very out of character for him. It seemed to Ben that his parents had held in all their feelings about his condition until just now, when they apparently perceived their son was not being treated with proper respect or care. They'd gone to such lengths to smooth his transition from Harley Rehab and now they were in no mood for him to be hassled.

"I think it'll be okay," Ben said, his palms sweating, trying to keep the lid on an eruption he hoped would subside. "It's only, you know, a formality, I'm sure. Let's wait until after the meeting to see what will happen," Ben said, reversing roles, assuming the grown-up assignment.

"Well, it sure better be okay," Jacob said, still simmering. "I'll talk to Sidney Segal before the meeting to get his advice."

"Getting Sidney involved doesn't seem like a good idea," Sophie said. "I agree with Ben. I think we ought to wait until to see how the meeting goes before we go off half-cocked and get Sidney involved. I like him, but he's a lawyer and lawyers tend to muddy the waters a lot."

"Dad," Ben said, also concerned that Jacob was rushing to judgment. "I don't want Segal involved unless we see a problem. We don't know that yet. Let's wait until after I meet." They all relaxed and agreed that they would be patient.

"How is Uncle Abraham?" Ben asked, after the conversation paused.

"About the same," Jacob said. "The last time I saw him he looked tired, but not in pain. He said to give you a hug for him."

Ben choked back a sob as his mind turned away from his own troubles to the challenges his uncle was facing.

"You know what he told me about the medical school? He said there's no way they won't let me finish. They're medical doctors whose mission in life is to help people. So, I'm keeping that in mind. Besides, I'm, what, three-fourths of a doctor already. I'm one of a hundred doctors-to-be in this class. The medical school can't afford to allow even one of us not to graduate, not with what they've already invested in us."

"I hadn't thought of it that way," Sophie said. "That makes sense to me. Very reassuring."

The dinner ended on that positive note. They went to Ben's room and played cards listening to the Boston Symphony concert on the radio until it was time for bed.

~~~

The meeting was set for ten in the morning on Tuesday. Jacob and Sophie took Ben. They got there early to help get him out of the car and into the office. They were greeted by a middle-aged woman with pince-nez glasses, a serious face. She told them that she'd tell the committee they were there. It wasn't long before she motioned Ben to come to the meeting room. He wheeled his chair through the open door and saw four men in the room.

"Good morning, Mr. Levinson, I'm Tim Garvey, Assistant Dean for Student Affairs. Let me introduce the members of the Committee: Dr. Philip Beecher, from Biochemistry, Dr. Daniel Crawford, from the Department of Internal Medicine, and Dr. Harry West, Assistant Professor of Pediatrics.

"Our purpose today is to determine the best course of action for you. Let me say first that there is no
~~~

question about your continuation as a student. What we need to do is see how we can best assist you."

Ben let out an audible sigh of relief.

"We've gathered information from a variety of places: the inpatient units you've been on, Harley Rehabilitation Unit, and we've talked with your medical providers. All have told us of your remarkable attitude and resilience. So, today we want to hear first-hand as to how you feel."

Ben's tension melted away. His grip on the wheelchair loosened, the stiffness in his neck muscles relaxed, and the twitch in his eye went away.

"I'm feeling rather good, all things considered," he said. "And I have to say, so relieved to hear what you just told me.

"I'm anxious to get back to seeing patients. I learned a lot *being* a patient. I think it will make me a better doctor. Also, I've kept up with my studies by reading my textbooks and lecture notes some of my fellow students have sent me.

"I'm curious to find out how to navigate the rest of my medical school and prepare for internship. By the way, I want to go into pediatrics," looking at Dr. West, "after I spent my rotation there. It may seem odd since the rotation in pediatrics is where I got polio that I would still choose that field, but I loved my interaction with the kids and felt most at home there. And because of my illness, my eyes were opened to people suddenly challenged by the loss of physical and mental functions. I think this is particularly true in pediatrics. I think I've found my mission.

"So, when can I come back?" he finally blurted.

What was first seen as an austere group of inquisitors now seemed like a group of supportive colleagues. They all smiled when he asked that, and Mr. Garvey replied,

"Soon as you feel you're ready. We must arrange for the internal medicine service to fit you into their care team. We have an occupational therapist advising us on planning for your smooth inclusion. The hospital is only just beginning to understand that physically limited people have a lot to contribute to medical care. An anonymous donor has offered to provide substantial help to make sure you get needed transportation and other assistance in negotiating any physical challenges you'll face."

Ben felt like kicking himself for ever doubting that he would be blocked from continuing his chosen field. Or that he'd been ignored. An anonymous donor pitching in! Who could that be? He could hardly wait to tell his parents and Abraham. He left the room with a broad smile on his face. Sophie and Jacob saw that smile and knew that all was well.

Chapter 12

Sandra

"Ben?"

"Yeah, who's this?"

"Sandra."

"What a surprise!" Ben said, taken completely off-balance by her out-of-the blue call. He hadn't recognized her voice, but that was understandable; he hadn't heard from her in over two years.

"I've been meaning to call for a while but felt funny about it," Sandra said. "I heard you were in a hospital and all, but I didn't know how you'd take it if I called."

Ben's mind went in reverse, with memories flooding over him, but he forced himself back to real time.

"Glad you called, Sandra," he replied cautiously. "What do you know about, um, my illness?"

"I heard you had polio, but that's about all I know."

"That's right, polio. Who told you?"

"Well, word gets around. I don't remember where I heard it," she said in a barely audible voice. "Are you okay now?"

"Yeah, I'm okay. I'm at home. Taking a little time off to get better."

"Are you still a med student?" she said, circling around, trying to have a real conversation but getting no help from Ben.

"Yes, as a matter of fact, I just met with people at the medical school. I'm going back to my hospital rotation in a couple of weeks.

"So, what are you doing with yourself?" Ben asked.

"Oh, I'm still at the Conservatory, doing musical composition and conducting. They tell me I'm wasting my time taking conducting since there aren't any women conductors. But I enjoy conducting so much."

Ben bit his tongue before he replied to this. He still nursed angry feelings from when she broke off their relationship, even though they'd had conflicts. Even then, he'd chafed at her need to be in charge. Her professed love of conducting reminded him of her penchant for control. He was tempted to tell her that was the reason she liked conducting so much. Instead, he said, "I'm glad you stuck with your music. Are you still playing piano?"

"Oh yeah, can't give that up. I pick up a few bucks playing at weddings, birthdays, Bar Mitzvahs and even funerals. Sometimes I sing, too."

Ben couldn't tell where this conversation was headed, and carefully chose every word, wary of what might come next. Sandra had always had a way of looking for something to be indignant about in everything he said.

"So, could I come and see you?" Sandra asked.

He froze. Should he tell her what to expect? She apparently didn't know any details about his illness or his paralysis. If he didn't tell her in advance, how would she take it when she saw him? Would she be angry that he hadn't forewarned her? He decided he had to tell her now and brave the consequences.

"I have to tell you more about my polio," he began. Searching for a way into the revelation about his paralysis, he said, "Remember President Roosevelt?"

"Yeah, he had polio. I remember vaguely that he used a wheelchair. What's that have to do with you?" A short pause. "Oh, no. Don't tell me that. You're not in a wheelchair, are you?" As the reality sunk in, she said, "Oh Ben, I'm so sorry. I didn't know the whole story, you know, about your illness." She broke off and the line went dead. Sandra came back on the line and said again, "Ben, I am so terribly sorry."

"Sandra. Listen. I don't want your pity, but I couldn't let you come here without warning you what you'd find. That kind of surprise shouldn't happen." *Should I head her off? Give her a way out to avoid the visit?*

"So, if you decide not to come, I'll understand. Considering all that has gone on between us, it's perfectly reasonable and understandable for you not to come."

"I still want to see you, Ben. We left too many things unresolved. I'm not asking to resume our relationship, but I want to at least be friends."

Ugh, that old thing about a former lover wanting to be "just friends."

"I'd like to be friends, too," Ben said, *since I can't be a sexual being anymore.* "Come when you can. I'm here most of the time but call to let us know when you're coming. You know Sophie. You and she really got along. She'll most likely be here when you come."

"How about now? I'm free today but have stuff to do for the next few days. Would today around two be alright for you?"

Ben drew in a deep breath. *So typical of Sandra. Taking charge. This is so precipitous. But might as well do it right away instead of obsessing about it.*

"Sure. Come to the kitchen door and Sophie will let you in." After he said that, he wondered what Sophie would think.

Sandra Robinson first attracted Ben's attention at a Dunster House party in his sophomore year at college. He was captivated, watching her in intense conversation with one of his house mates. After some initial hesitation, he sat down beside her, gazing at her as she continued talking and was, as he told it later, "smitten." Here she was, a feisty, petite brunette with a figure that attracted attention from all testosterone-driven males within 100 feet of her. Eschewing lipstick and mascara, her natural beauty was bewitching. Ben fell for her, hard.

He'd started seeing her regularly, halfway through college thinking that this relationship was the "real thing." But their romance developed only gradually. She was initially uninterested in him, this introspective pre-med kid. But as time went on and Ben persisted, she awakened to his sincerity, guilelessness, and essential goodness.

Their interest in one another built slowly while hiking together, attending Red Sox and Celtics games, stage plays and concerts, both rock and classical. They went often to Symphony Hall where Sandra had a student pass. Ben had learned to appreciate classical music from both his parents, who, in their childhoods in Germany were regulars at concerts in northern Germany. Once, he and Sandra were thrilled seeing Charles Munch conduct the Boston Symphony Orchestra's performance of Debussy's La Mer.

Sandra bonded with him around classical music while she studied at the Conservatory. Ben watched her first piano recital at Jordan Hall, falling in love even more as she performed Bach partitas flawlessly. Mutual interest in music became a major link in their romantic attachment.

He was in the middle of his first grueling year of medical school when fracture lines in their relationship began to appear. She accused him of ignoring her, and perhaps he had, in his preoccupation with dissection of his cadaver and the fascination of the wonders of biochemistry. She complained that his "new mistress" -- medical school -- had become the center of his universe, to the detriment of everything else, especially her. This was truer than Ben wanted to admit, and heated arguments about this led inexorably to an unpleasant last dinner together at Grendel's Den, where Sandra announced unceremoniously that she wanted out. And like most things with Sandra, when she decided something, there was no turning back. Ben was crushed, angry and surprised, all at the same time, never having a major failure in his young life.

As he mulled over the painful remembrance of this loss, he said, "Mom, guess who's coming to see me. Before you wrack your brain, I'll tell you: Sandra."

She frowned and said, "Why? She feeling guilty that she broke up with you? I'm still mad at her for throwing you over." She looked at Ben for a clue as to how he was reacting to the prospect of her coming to see him in his present condition. "How am I supposed to relate to her?"

"Just be pleasant, Mom. That all was a long time ago. She may be a different person now. I sure am. I'm willing to forgive her. She said she wanted to be friends. Holding a grudge only hurts the one hanging onto it, you always told me that."

"I'll do my best," Sophie said. Thinking about it, she said "Well, I got along pretty well with her, so I'll simply be the way I always was with her."

Both Ben and Sophie scampered around the kitchen and Ben's room, picking up discarded papers and magazines from the floor, Sophie quickly making Ben's bed, sniffing around the bathroom, opening the window to clear the air. Sophie dashed upstairs to change clothes. Ben checked to be sure he'd shaved that morning. Sandra had always disliked stubble on his face. Sophie came downstairs and said, "Do you remember whether she liked tea or coffee? Or soft drinks?"

"Probably tea. We have some Cokes in the refrig in case she wants that. Don't bother with anything else. It's just after lunch." Both were more anxious about Sandra's visit than either would admit.

Near two o'clock, a knock came at the kitchen door. Sophie took a deep breath and moved deliberatively toward the door.

"Hi, Mrs. Levinson," Sandra said quietly. "So good to see you. Thanks for letting me come."

"Welcome, Sandra. Good to see you too," offering her hand. "Come on in, have a seat. I'll call Ben." She disappeared into his room.

Ben wheeled into the kitchen, slightly nudging the wall as he came. Seeing Sandra brought a tsunami of memories, only some of them good. She looked the same as that first evening at the Dunster house and seeing her evoked the same erotic feeling he'd had then. First love never dies.

"Hi," was all he could think to say.

"Hi, yourself," Sandra said.

"You look great," he said, gripping the rails on his wheelchair with more force than necessary. "Wanna see where I live?" he chuckled.

"Sure. Can I give you a kiss?"

Bert blushed like a fifteen-year-old but managed to form the words, "help yourself."

Sandra came to the wheelchair, kneeled by his side, turned his head toward hers, and kissed him fully on the mouth. He was surprised to feel a stirring in his groin, and soon he was aroused fully. He didn't know what to do, so he said with a broad smile, "You haven't lost your touch." He then quickly turned his chair around and said, "Follow me, I'll show you around my pad."

"Sandra, would you like tea or coffee?" Sophie said as they headed toward Ben's room, not fully understanding what had just happened.

"No thanks, Sophie, I just had a cup with lunch."

Ben was excited that his capacity to respond sexually had not, after all, been lost, but was glad it had subsided. He proceeded to show Sandra all his contraptions for moving about as he jabbered away, demonstrating Rube Goldberg devices he'd rigged up for various tasks. Sophie was gratified to hear them laughing in Ben's room. She knew she should leave them alone as they embarked on their newfound "friendship."

Sandra didn't linger long. After Ben wound down showing off his paraphernalia, they had a long kiss goodbye and Sandra promised to return when she could stay longer. Ben was exhausted and hoisted himself into bed for a long nap and a dream in which he and Sandra were hiking along a segment of the Appalachian Trail in New Hampshire, hoping to reach Greenleaf before rain came. The clouds were threatening to behold, but Ben knew that Greenleaf had a hut they could stay in overnight if the expected storm made it necessary.

When the rains came, they were already cuddling in a room in the hut. Ben nuzzled his head into Sandra's neck, and it wasn't long until they were both undressed and making love. Thunder failed to deter their ardor, in fact made it more heated.

When Ben opened his eyes, he took in a different room. He squinted, trying to reorient to an awake state, as the light of day was fading in his room at home. The pleasurable glow of his dream dimmed to a cold reality of being alone, without Sandra, and disabled. He stifled deep sobs of despondency.

Chapter 13

Ellen Jankowicz

"Remember the med school got an occupational therapist to advise us on what we need at home for mobility assistance? Well, I just heard from her. She's coming today at 2. Her name is Ellen Jankowicz," Ben said to his parents over breakfast.

"Oh, I gotta be here for that. I'll come home after lunch," Jacob said. "That's exciting. What kind of things did she mention?"

"Two main areas: transportation and home equipment. I think she'll be pleased with the things you did already, Dad. Not sure what else I'm gonna need. That hospital bed you got is perfect for me.

"Driving a car, though, is my major concern. The Suburban needs some modifications or whatever you call it, so I can drive it," Ben said. He paused, shaking his head. "I can't get over that car. It's the biggest one I've ever seen! You could live in that thing."

Ellen Jancowicz came at two o'clock on the dot. She swept into the house carrying pictures and manuals of illustrations for home health aides. She moved around

Ben's room like a ballerina, her eyes darting from bed to chairs to bathroom, with approving nods when she saw all that Jacob had accomplished.

"Wow, you're way ahead of me! Look at what you've already done! I'm impressed!" she exclaimed.

Jacob smiled, proud that this dynamo of a woman approved of all he'd done, but he was anxious to hear what further things were needed.

"I have a suggestion," Sophie said. "Why don't we meet around the dining room table?"

"Good idea!" enthused Ellen. They all gathered around the table, directing their attention to Ellen, who clearly was going to be the star of this show. She passed around various manuals on equipment to the three of them.

"I think the place to start is about mobility and the activities of daily living, or ADL. Getting in and out of bed for someone with no leg strength requires what we call a transfer trapeze. These come in various design, but when you get one, don't go cheap. You need a sturdy device that will support the demand put on it.

"How much do you weigh, Ben?"

"Last time I was weighed in Harley I was 160. But I'm gaining weight with Mom's cooking."

"You're lighter than most, but still, I'd advise getting a strong trapeze. That's a must to get in and out of bed to do anything. I see that you've got all you need in the bathroom.

"Then there's the issue of the wheelchair. Folding chairs have been available since the 1930's and I'd advise getting one of these for easy transport. The wheelchair you're in, Ben, is a better chair, but not easily transported. That brings up another issue: a good wheelchair at your destination. You can use the folding chair, but for all-day use it's not very comfortable. So, if you can have one like this at the hospital, that would be ideal.

"Any questions?"

"A few simple ones. For example, how do I get myself positioned in the driver's seat of our car, and how do I get the wheelchair in and out of the Suburban? How do I drive it with no legs? How do I get a license to drive while handicapped? When I hear answers to these questions, I'll feel a lot better."

"It's not hard to see your priorities, Ben," she laughed. "But to be honest: there are several steps to take before you're ready to drive. Have you been fitted for leg braces?"

"No." It began to sink in that this was not going to be as easy or fast as he'd hoped.

"Braces on your legs, locked into the vertical position, allows you to stand before you swing your body into the cab of the car. Getting in and out of the car from your wheelchair also requires strong arms and shoulders. So, you must build up your arm strength by doing lots of exercises. Lifting weights is the simplest way to do this. You can lift weights while in bed or in your chair. As you progress, other exercises can be added, including swimming."

Turning to Jacob, she said, "Do you know any welders?"

"Welders? No, but I can find one, I'm sure. Why?"

"You need a strong bar welded above and inside the driver's door so Ben can use it to pull himself up into the driver's seat. Ben, this is also why you need to build up your arm and upper body strength. You're gonna need it.

"I'll show you a few tricks and suggest some things about stowing your wheelchair. But let's go first to your other questions about driving. By the way, I saw your Suburban outside before I came in. Looks like a great vehicle. It will be just the ticket for this endeavor. Does it have an automatic transmission?"

Jacob answered quickly, "Oh yes, that was one of the things I made clear to the car salesman."

"Nowadays, automatic transmissions are more standard in cars, the Hydramatic® being the most widely available," Ellen said. "The other good news is that just this year a man named Alan Ruprecht, an inventor and engineer, created the Drive-Master®, a push-pull hand control of accelerator and brake. Ruprecht also had polio and is paralyzed like you, Ben. That motivated him to invent the Drive-Master®. And now that we have automatic transmissions, it's much easier to adapt vehicles like yours to drive using these hand controls. See the pictures I brought? These let the driver use the right hand to steer and the left to control the accelerator and brake: push to brake and pull to accelerate. A round knob attached to the steering wheel lets the driver turn the steering wheel easily. I can show you some models of this back at Harley when you come for therapy. I'm not sure if Drive-Masters® are available yet in Boston, but I know they are in New York." She looked around at her attentive audience. "How're we doin'?"

"I'm sure glad I live now, with all these gadgets," Ben said. "But I'm still curious. How do I get my chair in and out of the Suburban?"

"I'm coming to that. In the old days the few people who designed cars for disabled drivers thought that you should just be able to wheel the chair into the vehicle. There was this box-like vehicle called the Invacar® allowing a person to drive while they were seated in their wheelchair after they moved it into the chassis. Terribly unsafe things, and never available in the States, thank heavens.

"So, to answer your question, until you establish your routine, you'll need help getting in and out of the car. After you get out of the wheelchair and pull yourself up into the driver's seat, you'll need someone to put the wheelchair away. This is why you need more than one chair. And then when you get where you're going, you'll need someone to unload the chair in the car and bring it around to you at the driver's door. I'll help you figure out how to get in and out of the chair and into the van and the reverse of that when you get to your destination."

"We can get Ben into the car here," Jacob said.

"I'm also able to retrieve the wheelchair after he's in the car," Sophie volunteered.

"So there needs to be a wheelchair in the Suburban that can be unloaded at your destination, Ben," Ellen said. "I'll explain how that's done.

"We'll make it easy for everyone by rigging up a ramp that will slide in and out of the rear end of the Suburban. The guys at Harley are used to these kinds of assignments. So, with a ramp, you won't have to do much lifting," she laughed. "Well, I gotta get outta here. I'm late for my next appointment."

"Before you go, one other quick question," Ben said. "How do I get a license to drive?"

"Don't worry, I'll see to that when the time comes," she said. "Usually, with a regular driving license and a recommendation from a professional driving instructor the Registry of Motor Vehicles will issue a license." After gazing around at the family, she went on, "I don't want to leave on a negative note, but I must tell you one more thing."

Jacob, Sophie, and Ben all exchanged glances, wondering what this seemingly ominous statement would be.

"You can't rush this process." Looking at Jacob and Sophie, she said, "Plan on someone driving Ben for a while before we start his solo flights. Ben, I can tell you're anxious to get into that behemoth of a car, rev it up and go, but there are numerous things you'll face as you go into this new phase of your life. You can handle them, I have no doubt about that, but try to be patient and not rush them.

"Well, it's been a great pleasure meeting all of you and I look forward to working with you as we solve all these things together." She gathered her purse, waved, said goodbye and left with the same dispatch as she had come.

After they thanked her, Ben looked at his parents and they all nodded in agreement that, wow, this was one extraordinary woman.

Chapter 14

Abraham's Note

"I'll find a welder to install that pull-bar for the van. And while I'm downtown I'll get some barbells and other exercise equipment," Jacob said to Ben. "Maybe I'll join you in exercises. I could use some workouts. I guess leg braces are something that Harley can advise us about. They'll probably have to be fitted to you and made to order. Anything else to put on my list?"

"Did Ellen tell us where we can find information about Drive-Master®? We need to get that installed soon," Ben said, clearly anxious to get this show on the road.

"Are you and Sophie going to practice getting you into the car?" Jacob asked.

"We may have to wait for a ramp for the chair. But we can start experimenting," Sophie said. Just then the phone rang, and Sophie ran to answer it.

"Levinson's. Yes. Oh, no!" she gasped. "Here, let me have you talk to my husband," handing the receiver to Jacob.

"Yes. When? God almighty!" Listening, nodding, jotting a few things down on the notepad next to the phone. "What do you need me to do?" Another pause. "I'll get back to you. Thank you."

Jacob sat down hard on the chair near the phone, feeling faint. Scenes from his childhood, when he idolized his much older brother, flashed through his mind.

Ben knew it was about his uncle.

"Bad news," Jacob, now calming himself and aware of his role in the family, said evenly. "Abraham died during the night. The nurse found him this morning when she came to start her shift. Worried about how he looked the night before, she told him then that she could stay with him for the night, but he insisted she go home to be with her family. So typical of him. But she couldn't have done anything, I'm sure.

"She asked me to call the funeral home in Cambridge. She said he'd left detailed instructions on his desk, knowing his time was short." Jacob was wrestling with his emotions but maintained his equanimity.

Sophie was already crying as she moved to comfort Jacob, and to be comforted. Ben closed his eyes, chin dropping to his chest. But he couldn't cry. *I knew this was coming, maybe that's why I'm not crying,* he thought. He stayed immobile, almost catatonic, as though his own body had died in sympathy.

Jacob took charge in his business-like mode, made the necessary calls, and left for Cambridge without another word. Sophie looked at Ben.

"I know how much you loved him, Ben. I grew to love him too. I'm sorry."

"I do love him and will miss him. So much." He looked at Sophie as she dried her tears. "I need time for this to sink in," he said. "I don't want to talk about it now, if you don't mind."

Sophie nodded, kissed Ben on his cheek, and busied herself with cleaning up the breakfast dishes.

Jacob returned from Cambridge with the list of instructions Abraham had left on his desk. He wanted to be buried in the Jewish cemetery in Newton, after a private funeral service at the Levine Funeral Home and it "should occur within two days of my death," according to his instructions. Thankfully, this left little for Jacob to do.

Abraham left the address of a lawyer in Central Square who had prepared a simple will, leaving everything in Abraham's modest estate to United Jewish Appeal-Federation of New York. Jacob went to the library and called Bernie Weiner, Abraham's friend and colleague at MIT. Bernie received the news quietly, unsurprised at the death since he had seen Abraham a few days before and recognized then that he was close to death. These plans were typical of Abraham's careful strategies, always considerate of others, taking care the family was not inconvenienced in any way.

Ben noticed that on his return from Cambridge, Jacob moved and talked slowly, apparently numbed by his older brother's death. He stood limp as Sophie gave him a hug, seemingly unable to focus on the present. He gradually threw off this ennui and returned from his preoccupation with mortality. He looked at Ben, whose eyes had widened in surprise at his father's uncharacteristic torpid aspect and handed him a white envelope.

"This was on his desk. It's addressed to you," he said in a serious tone.

Ben reached out and grasped the envelope. Only his name was on the outside. His hands shook as he carefully opened it.

My Dear Ben,

My life has been satisfying in many ways. I have the usual regrets of an old man, but I am at peace, recognizing the truth that "to err is human, to forgive divine," so I have forgiven myself of mistakes I made along the way.

There are innumerable things I had hoped to discuss further with you, but your illness and mine conspired to prevent those conversations. I'm sorry.

I first met you when you were ten years old. Even then, in my eyes, you had a quality of spirit that set you apart. Your mind and heart are in synchrony and harmony. You have a special capacity to understand and identify with another person's troubles and pleasures. This, and your intellectual curiosity, will make you a complete physician. These things were evident early on.

You have been afflicted with a terrible disease. This threatens to rob you of your mission of healing the physical, mental, and emotional sickness of your future patients.

This must not happen.

You are alive and vibrant, and I see you living a long and useful life. You have already demonstrated your strength of character and resilience. You will rise above this dreadful setback and give the world your caring hands and skills. I don't know and I doubt you know yet what trail you will carve out, but I know you will be a role model to all who have you in their lives.

As I cross into the unknown, I hope you will carry some memory of me and think of the many ideas and thoughts we have shared. I have gained a measure of understanding from my hardships, and I believe your hardships will likewise yield wisdom to you. I hope some of the things I have told you will be helpful in the future.

You have been as a son to me, and I thank you for being in my world.

With warmth and love,
Uncle Abraham

"Would you like to hear this?" Ben asked.

Jacob and Sophie nodded. Ben took a deep breath, gathered himself, and read to them in a wavering voice. When he was finished, he looked at his parents and tears that previously were trapped inside now came in a torrent. Ben cried unashamedly as his parents rushed to his side, joining him in a mutual release of grief at the family's loss.

Abraham's funeral was simple and of short duration as he desired. Bernie Weiner, his MIT boss and benefactor, the family, and a few people from Weiner's laboratory attended. Bernie spoke about his friendship with Abraham.

"I've known Abraham since our days together at medical school in Germany. His empathy for other people was evident to all, even at that early part of his life. He went into medical practice. I left Germany because I was interested in research, but I never forgot Abraham. When he called after his arrival in Boston in 1939, wondering about working with me, I had no hesitation in offering him a job in my department at MIT. His help with my research was immeasurable and his name will appear on several scientific papers from my lab. But even more than that, I was thrilled to be reunited with one of the most talented and caring physicians I've ever known. I, and all the others who knew and worked with him, will miss him immensely."

Jacob, Sophie, and Ben each told of their love for Abraham, with tears and tremulous voices. The service was short and modest, like the life Abraham had lived. The family would cherish his memory and forever be grateful for the gift of knowing him.

Chapter 15

Accident

In November 1952, Dwight D. Eisenhower won the Presidency of the United States. He was the world-famous Supreme Commander of the Allied Expeditionary Force who oversaw the 1944 Normandy invasion and ushered in the Allies' victory in the European campaign. His fame was complemented by his down-to-earth personality and his campaign slogan, "I Like Ike." He won in a landslide.

Ben didn't dislike Eisenhower although he was mildly disappointed. He leaned toward Adlai Stevenson because of his erudition and intellect. Although Ben followed both campaigns closely, he couldn't vote because voting in Brookline took place on the third floor of an old building with no access for disabled people. Another frustration of everyday life to deal with.

His rehabilitation was going well, his upper body strength improving with exercise, and he was mastering his transfer from bed to chair, from chair to car. Most important, he moved comfortably in his wheelchair on hospital rounds. By the end of the day, however, he was exhausted and always fell into a deep sleep. However, on his days off, he avidly followed American League baseball scores. This summer, his beloved Red Sox were nineteen games behind the hated Yankees who went on to the World Series, facing their crosstown rivals, "dem bums," otherwise known as the Brooklyn Dodgers. The Yankees were trying to make it four consecutive World Series championships. When he had time, Ben was glued to the radio and devoured the sports section of the Boston Globe following each game. Because he supported two teams -- the Boston Red Sox and any team that beat the Yankees -- he naturally was rooting for the Dodgers to win this World Series.

But it was not to be. The Yankees won in seven, with three veteran pitchers, Allie Reynolds, called "Chief" because of his Native American heritage, was the winning pitcher in two games. Vic Raschi and Eddie Lopat each had one win. Yogi Berra was the catcher in all the games, a star both behind the plate and in the batter's box. Mickey Mantle hit a key home run in one game and Berra hit two. Ben couldn't help but admire the Bronx Bombers for their grit and determination even though he was unhappy with the outcome.

1952 was also notable in that there were over 57,000 cases of polio in the United States, 3145 with fatal outcomes, and 21,269 cases of mild to severe paralysis, more than ever before. Ben was in the smallest group, those with severe paralysis. But he felt grateful to be alive and able to pursue his dream of becoming a doctor.

Although Ben learned, with his parents' help, how to get in and out of the car, he was impatient for the Drive-Master® system to be delivered and installed in the Suburban. A retractable ramp with a weighted block and tackle that worked with a pulley was now in its cargo compartment so his 45-pound monster wheelchair could be rolled in and out. Jacob helped Ben into the car at home, Sophie drove him to the hospital and hospital orderlies lifted him out of the car into his wheelchair. He insisted on propelling his wheelchair to the wards by hand and used his cane to press the elevator buttons.

Still, Ben was getting antsy to start driving himself. Sophie admitted she'd be nervous riding in the front passenger seat while Ben was on a steep learning curve of navigating the crowded streets between Chestnut Hill and the hospital. But trouper that she was, she agreed to do it.

Just before the holiday season began, the Drive-Master® arrived. Accompanying the equipment were instructions on installation, together with the name of a driving instructor in Boston who coached prospective users how to operate it safely. Jacob found a mechanic to install it and called the driving instructor, Avery Streeter, to schedule an appointment.

Ben was thrilled at the prospect of being freed from his dependency on his parents for transportation.

Avery Streeter was an athletic fifty-three-year-old woman with a calm demeanor and complete familiarity with the equipment. She and Ben hit it off from the start. It took only a few lessons until he was ready to take his first run, with Avery in the passenger seat and Jacob and Sophie leaning over from the back seat to watch.

Ben was a quick study. With only a few more lessons he was ready to do a solo run without Avery in the car.

"I'm going with you, you know," Sophie said as Ben settled into the driver's seat. "I need to get used to riding with you. I won't nag you, I promise."

"Sure you want to put your life in my hands?" Ben asked, with a laugh.

"I'll try not to make you nervous," Sophie said, trying hard not to show her own anxiety.

"So, what about me? Don't I get to come too?" Jacob said with a smile.

"This is a family celebration, so hop on in, Dad! I can see the headlines now: 'Entire family dies in a spectacular automobile crash,'" Ben quipped. He had acquired what was known as "gallows humor" in the hospital to offset the oft-seen tragedies of disease and death.

Sophie and Jacob said in unison, "Oh, Ben, don't talk that way!"

But the solo drive went well. The next step was taken in the morning with only Sophie aboard. It went without a hitch.

The transport guys at the hospital gave up a cheer when they saw Ben driving into the drop-off area where they always met.

"Congratulations, Bennie!" Alonzo and Raffy said in unison when arrived. Ben was exhilarated when he was helped down from the driver's seat.

"This is a new angle to get you out," Alonzo laughed. "Sort of a mirror image of what we've been doing," referring to assisting him from the passenger side.

In time, Ben got comfortable with the routine of getting out of the car without help. He established a routine: with his hands, he lifted his flaccid legs toward the open door of the car, then locked his knee braces in place so his legs were straight. Sliding his body down from the driver's seat, he planted his feet on the ground, steadying himself with his now strong arms. With crutches he maneuvered around to the cargo compartment and pulled the ramp, then brought his wheelchair down to the ground. Once it was braked and in position, he sat down in it, unlocked his knee braces, lifted his legs into the foot saddles and jerked on the pulley to roll the ramp back into the car. Grabbing the circular handles on the wheelchair, he rolled into the hospital. After a few days this ritual became smoother.

About a week into driving with the new gadgetry he was feeling confident. But that confidence was short-lived.

"Benji, watch out for that car coming out of that driveway!" Sophie screamed on their way to the hospital the next day. Too late. He plowed into the sedan with a sickening loud thud, damaging the back door, rear wheel, and fender of the other car. The driver leaped out red-faced, waving his arms wildly.

"God damned, stupid sonofabitch!" he screamed as he strode toward the Suburban, tearing open Ben's door and grabbing his arm, yanking him from the car. Ben crashed hard onto the ground with the man standing over him, yelling, "Why don't you look where you're going, you stupid kid!"

Sophie leaped out of her side of the car, ran around behind the car, knelt beside Ben, screaming at the man, "You backed right into us! Don't just stand there yelling at him, help me get this boy up off the ground!"

She looked at Ben lying on the ground and began to cry. Ben was more angry than hurt, as he looked up at his mother and the man glaring at each other. He sat up and screamed at the man, "You should look where you're going, you fucking idiot! We could have all been killed and it's your fault! Help me up, for Chrissake."

By then, the man, who had momentarily discharged his anger, began to grasp that Ben was unable to walk and that he'd just attacked a disabled man. He leaned over and pulled Ben up to a sitting position, realizing that he had no function in his legs. He and Sophie got him back into the car.

"I didn't realize you were a cripple," he said, condescendingly. Ben was fuming as he looked at him.

"I may be crippled but I'm not stupid and careless," he spit out, still furious this had happened, especially during his first week of driving.

A police siren signaled the approach of a cruiser. Someone had seen the accident and called the police. Sophie by now had collected herself, but still was enraged at this aggressive jerk who not only caused a bad accident but had attacked her disabled son. The policeman walked toward the three of them.

"Who wants to tell me what happened here?" he said.

Sophie spoke up immediately. "This" -- she could hardly speak -- "person," she sputtered, "was backing out of his driveway, paying no attention to the street. No way my son could stop without hitting him. We ploughed into the back of his car. Then this guy," she sneered, "jumps out of his car, completely out of control, pulls the car door open and drags my son onto the ground. He should be arrested for assault and battery!"

"And you," the cop said, trying to stay non-judgmental as he turned to face the man, who was busy inspecting the damage to his car, "what's your name, and what's your side of the story, sir?"

"I'm Carl Krebs," and pointing to Ben he said, "That kid's a cripple and couldn't control his car. He can't even walk let alone drive. There ought to be a law against letting cripples like that drive. He shoulda' stopped when he saw me trying to get outta' my drive. This is a busy street, and I always have trouble getting out. Nobody gives you a break."

The cop turned to Ben. "Is it true you're crippled?"

"That isn't the term I use," Ben said, irritated by this word and by the colossal mean-spiritedness of Krebs. "My legs are paralyzed secondary to polio. But that isn't why the accident happened. I drive a specialized car with assists built in. This guy just backed, willy-nilly, out of his driveway. Not my fault. The accident has nothing to do with my paralysis. Then this animal came and pulled me out of the car, landing me on the ground. That's inexcusable. He was in a rage. I'm lucky I'm not badly injured."

"Well, in any case, you," looking at Ben, "need to be seen at the hospital for an evaluation," the officer said. "And I need all your names and other information. I'll call an ambulance for you," nodding to Ben, "and a wrecker," looking at Krebs, "to tow your car away. The rear wheel is jammed under the fender, so it's un-roadworthy."

He took all the needed information from them and sat down in his cruiser to make the calls. Krebs stormed back into his house, still fuming, wholly unrepentant.

The Suburban wasn't damaged at all, being more tank than automobile. The policeman allowed Sophie to drive Ben to the hospital with instructions for the staff to call Officer Timilty, the cop at the scene, for details about the accident. He was examined promptly, X-rays taken of his head, back, legs and arms, which showed that he was unharmed except for a bruised buttock where he'd fallen, and then he was discharged. Ben insisted on going to the wards and joining his colleagues for rounds, even if late.

When Jacob heard about the details of the accident, he was nearly out of control.

"This time I am calling Stanley! I'm gonna sue that bastard Krebs and bring criminal charges for assault and battery on my son. I can't believe there are people like that roaming around in civilized society." He kept on ranting until even he grew tired of hearing his complaining.

Jacob called Stanley. After listening to the description of the accident and reviewing the benign hospital assessment of Ben's condition, he calmed Jacob down. He called Krebs, identifying himself as the family's lawyer and told him they were considering filing a lawsuit to see if that would have the desired effect. It did. Krebs said he'd pay for the damages to his car and Ben's ER visit costs if Stanley would back off and not file a suit.

Despite the emotional trauma from the accident, Sophie recognized that Ben was not at fault and decided reluctantly that he was ready to drive by himself. She insisted, however, that he call her each day as soon as he got to the hospital.

~~~

Despite missing nearly four months of school, the faculty decided that Ben could sit for the final exams of his junior year and enter his final year so he would graduate with his classmates. He used the time at home studying his medical textbooks and the lecture notes given to him by his classmates. Happily, he aced the final exams. He was elected to Alpha Omega Alpha, an honorary fraternity for high scholastic achievement in medical school. Now came his next major decision.
~~~

Chapter 16

Decisions

Now in the winter of his senior year, Ben had to decide where to go for internship and residency. His inclination was to stay put at Boston Pediatric Hospital if he could get into this highly competitive internship. He met with his advisor, Dr. Clifford Boyd, during the December holiday break.

"I advise everyone to go to a hospital dissimilar from the one they know from medical school. It gives you another venue, a different point of view, a different perspective on clinical medicine. It may look easier to stay here in familiar surroundings at Channing. But you should spread your wings, see other places," Dr. Boyd said.

"Am I getting a not-so-hidden message that I'd have trouble getting a slot here?"

"No, no, that's not what I'm saying at all. I give this advice to everyone graduating from this great medical school. But I believe that exposing yourself to other thinking enriches the mind."

"Where can I go where there would be any better faculty than here?"

"Plenty of places. Some people here are very parochial and think there is no better place in the universe for medical education, pure academic hubris in that. If you want to stay in Boston, apply also to Suffolk County Hospital across town. Ambulances bring many cases there from the inner city and you'll see a different palette of diseases and trauma. There are other hospitals in the area who also offer great internships."

Ben stole a glance out of the window and caught a glimpse of the familiar dome of Boston Pediatric Hospital. He felt a twinge of regret at the thought of leaving this place he'd known for nearly four years, for the unknown.

"I have a unique need to stay in Boston, you know," he said, returning to the moment. "My living space at home is ideal for my, um, disability." He always stumbled over that word. "Any place I intern needs to have wards and intern quarters that I can get in and out of without a big hassle. I mean, I don't expect any special privileges, but I have some specific needs. Plus, I know Boston," Ben explained. "But I heard that Suffolk County Hospital has a lot of deteriorating buildings. Is that true?"

"The buildings there are quite old, that's a fact. But there's an esprit de corps there, a dedication to serving the inner city's poor population that makes it a special place. I trained there and loved my time there."

"How hard is it to get in there?"

"Every internship in Boston is tough. Suffolk's no exception. But with your record here and strong recommendations from our faculty, which I'm sure you'll get, I think you stand a good chance. Give it a shot."

When Ben had dinner with Sophie and Jacob that night, he told them what Dr. Boyd had said.

"I don't know, Ben," Jacob said. He'd read newspaper articles describing chronic problems with Suffolk County Hospital, especially the county government's stingy funding for the place. "That's a tough neighborhood over there. The physical plant is a dump, from what I hear. Why can't you just apply to Boston Pediatric and be done with it?"

"Do they have parking and the kind of access you need there?" Sophie chimed in. "You know, can you get to elevators easily? I also worry about all those terrible cases there—gunshot wounds, stabbings, drunks, drug addicts, all that. I'd be worried about you there."

"I'd have to interview there, so I can check those things out. But it reminds me of the kind of neighborhood Uncle Abe served in Hamburg. He took care of the inner-city population and considered that his mission in life. He was in love with his community. I can see myself doing something like that," Ben said.

"The other thing is, I'm not sure I could get an internship at Boston Pediatric. It's one of the most desirable internships in the country. It's highly competitive."

"Nonsense, Ben," Jacob said. "You were elected to AOA and graduated near the top in your class. You're competitive with anybody. And they know you."

"Yeah, all true," Ben said. He knew this would be a hard sell. "But the mission at Suffolk is community-oriented and at Boston Pediatric the mission there tilts more to laboratory research, generation of new knowledge, and preparation of residents to go on to chairmanships in pediatric departments all over the country. All important, sure, but I want to take care of patients. And teach. Maybe do some clinical research, but bench research, uh-uh, just not my interest."

"But having Boston Pediatric on your resume, added to your Channing Medical School diploma, would almost guarantee a great future," Jacob said, ever the pragmatist.

"If you want private practice, you could probably find an already established doctor close to retirement who'd hire you on the spot. I think that's more desirable than what Abe did. He was penniless when he got here, remember? You wanna' live a good life or be Don Quixote?"

Ben realized that this would have to be his decision and his alone. His father would never fathom Abraham's devotion to his patients, his sense of mission. The two brothers were so unalike one would never know they had the same parents. But Ben also fully grasped and appreciated his parents' desire for his well-being and happiness. His mother was nervous, as she'd always been, about his safety, compounded now by his paralysis. His father understood the importance of making money, and devoted himself to that, a role in which he'd been highly successful. Ben had to admit he'd benefited greatly from his father's affluence and was immensely grateful to him for what he'd provided to him. But this was the second immense turning point in his life, the first being polio, a truly existential threat.

"I understand your concerns," Ben said. "I have some of these same feelings. Good questions and suggestions, too. I need more info about Suffolk. I'll get an interview there, look carefully at the place. Also need an interview at Boston Pediatric Hospital, even though I'm intimately acquainted, more than I wanted to be, with that hospital. And go from there. Big decisions ahead."

"Well, gather your information and we can talk about it more. When will you have your interviews?" Jacob asked quietly.

"Not for a while. I must wait until a certain date when we're allowed to make appointments. Not sure of that date yet."

~~~
~~~

Because neither of them knew about parking, Sophie took him to the Suffolk County Hospital in early January for his interview. He met Dr. Philip Andersen in the Mary Flannigan Pediatric Pavilion since he'd indicated his interest in pediatrics. Dr. Anderson was in his forties, slender and fit. His reddish-brown hair spilled over his forehead and Ben noticed his large blue eyes bulged slightly. *Could he have had Graves' disease?* The part of Ben's mind that loved to make diagnoses turned on as he looked at him. His quick pace as he wheeled Ben to the elevator supported Ben's opinion that he might have an overactive thyroid. After they were seated side by side on a couch in Dr. Andersen's third floor office Ben waited for him to start the interview.

"Welcome to County Hospital. Have you ever been here before?"

"No sir, never. Seems odd, though, since I was born and raised in Boston."

"You're the first local guy I've met since these current interviews have begun. Most applicants have been from elsewhere. So, I'm glad to meet you. Where do you live?"

"Chestnut Hill," Ben said, sheepishly, since it was such an elite suburb.

"I live two blocks from here, on Worcester Court. My wife and I bought one of those bowfront three-story buildings about five years ago and have been rehabbing it ever since. The bones of those old buildings are great, but restoration sure takes a long time and money."

He seems so easy to talk to. I like him already.

"I've looked over your curriculum vitae and I'm impressed. I've also been filled in about your paralytic polio. Needless to say, I'm sorry that came your way. So much of it this year.

"So, what can I tell you about County Hospital?"

Ben asked perfunctory questions about the patient load, types of patients, what night call was like, how busy they were, and other routine questions.

Since they were generic questions all applicants asked, Dr. Andersen handed him a sheet of paper with the answers.

"We've arranged for you to meet one of our residents who'll give you her view of the program. Better coming from her than from me, since she's living it. She'll also give you a tour. Are you applying for a straight pediatric internship or a rotating?"

"Any advice about that?"

"Depends on your level of certainty about pediatrics. If you know pediatrics is what you want, straight is the answer. If you're unsure, go the rotating route."

"Does it make any difference being accepted?" Ben laughed. "More applicants in one or the other?"

"No, we like either pathway. The number of applicants is usually about the same. But surgery is part of the rotating program, requires a lot of standing. How do you feel about that?"

"I never wanted to be a surgeon, even before polio. I always liked internal medicine, but like kids better. Much better. Sounds like I should do a straight peds internship."

"Okay. I'll put you in that applicant pile. Let me introduce you to Dr. Garrison."

They went to the seventh floor and Ben met Dr. Andrea Garrison who greeted him warmly with a handshake.

"Glad to meet you, Ben. I've heard a lot about you."

Ben wondered what she'd heard.

For the next hour, she took Ben from the top to the bottom of the Flannigan Building. Two of the floors were outpatient clinics, three were inpatient wards, the top floor was a large auditorium, "where we have weekly grand rounds and other conferences scattered through the week. We also have departmental parties up here."

Ben was impressed with the personalities and warmth of the people he met and found the physical plant not so bad after all. Andrea had taken him onto the wards where he saw some playful kids, some sleeping, some others crying for their mothers, but all being looked after by a caring nursing staff. He went to the pediatric intensive care unit, where he saw one three-month-old baby in coma because of a head injury allegedly sustained falling out of a fourth story window. Ben was puzzled. How could a baby that age, non-ambulatory, get to and fall out of a window?

"How could that happen? That kid couldn't possibly have fallen out of a window."

"That's right. The residents and the attending don't believe the story. They've already filed a report of suspected abuse, and the state Department of Social Services is investigating. This kid," nodding her head in the direction of another child, a toddler, "opened a cupboard door under the kitchen sink, found a container of bleach, took a swig of it, followed by screaming and retching. His mother brought him immediately to the emergency room, but the erosion from the bleach required a feeding tube to be inserted through his abdominal wall while the surgeons watch the esophagus with X-rays to see if it heals without scarring shut. If not, they're considering bringing up a loop of small intestine to replace the esophagus, a major procedure."

What cases they have here, Ben mused as they continued rounds: a case of lead poisoning, buttock skin burns bad enough for hospital care, a recovering case of bacterial meningitis, two cases of croup, one case of ruptured appendix. Amazing. Ben had read about these diseases only in textbooks but had not ever seen them in real kids. These were in addition to several cases of diarrhea and two cases of asthma, requiring oxygen, a case of a little girl with a sickle cell anemia pain crisis, and one other child with seizures.

"Thanks so much for this tour, Andrea. Really an eye-opener."

"Any questions?" she asked as she helped Ben navigate a hall with gurneys and wheelchairs, parked there for want of enough space.

"What do your on-call rooms look like? With my need for access in this wheelchair, I need to know I can get around."

"I'll take you to what we call the Ritz Hotel. It's pretty basic, but I think you'd be able to maneuver okay. It's clean, not too neat -- we're kind of preoccupied with other stuff and not so careful about all our personal things -- but it works for us. Bathrooms right there and, of course, the telephone, which we sometimes want to shove into the wastebasket," she laughed.

They took the elevator to the eighth floor, and she showed him the on-call rooms. *Not too bad*, thought Ben. *I can handle this. Can handle being on-call at night too.*

He left Suffolk County Hospital with a good feeling about it.

Chapter 17

A Chance Meeting

Half done, Ben thought. Next week, Boston Pediatric. *I don't really need a tour there. I know that place like my own house. Who'll interview me? Someone I know?*

Just like in old black and white movies where the day sheets of a desk calendar were shown fluttering away, carried off by an unseen wind, the next week flashed by. After parking his Suburban, he wheeled his chair under the ancient green dome of the Fenway Building and pushed the UP button at the elevator. The doors opened and Ben was startled when he saw Cathy Kelly emerging. She pulled up abruptly and cried out, "Ben! For heaven's sake, how are you? I've wondered about you so often, but I didn't know who to ask how you are doing."

Ben felt a red tide rushing up his cheeks as he gazed at her face, in his view a vision close to angelic, the same feeling he had when she came into his hospital room at the nadir of his illness. She was about five and a half feet tall, with roasted almond hair, dark emerald eyes, and high cheekbones in a statuesque face. Her shoulders were narrow with slender arms and small hands. She reminded Ben of Audrey Hepburn.

"Cathy," he stammered, "how are you?" was the best he could do.

"I'm fine, thanks," she said, also searching for words. "What are you doing here?"

"Headed for my internship interview, up on three," he said, then, "are you going to be around in an hour? I'd love to have a cup of coffee or tea with you."

"I wish I could, but I have something I've got to do downtown," she said, clearly disappointed. "But let me give you my phone number. I really want to catch up with you. Call me tonight?"

"Sure, um, by then I may even have a better idea about where I wanna go for internship, either here or at Suffolk County," fumbling his words. "So glad to have run into you. Talk to you later!"

He almost missed getting into the elevator in his excitement. As the doors were sliding together, he managed to squeeze into the elevator, alarming some of the other passengers.

"Sorry. I just saw an old friend and I forgot where I was going," he said, flushing with embarrassment.

Surprised that he was so stirred by seeing Cathy -- since he hardly knew her -- he was, nevertheless, inexorably drawn to her.

Hold on, he thought, remember your condition before you get all twitterpated. How many women want a man in a wheelchair?

The elevator dinged at the third floor, doors sliding open. He moved his chair out, turned right, and found Room 307. He knocked and the door was opened by a man, who was probably in his sixties, judging by his white hair, a slight stoop to his shoulders, and deep creases around his mouth and across his forehead. His penetrating bright blue eyes beneath his bushy eyebrows were impressive and a little frightening to Ben when he first saw him. But his deep voice and manner were reassuring, so Ben relaxed, shifting slightly in his not-so-comfortable wheelchair.

"Hello, I'm Dr. Caldwell. You would be Ben Levinson, right? Come in."

"Thanks. Yes, good to meet you," offering his hand.

Dr. Caldwell shook his hand, closed the door, and nodded toward the couch.

"I'll sit here on the couch. You can just stay there in your chair, okay? Have you liked Channing Medical School?" Dr. Caldwell asked.

What to say? He'd heard from some of his fellow students that some of these interviewers asked questions from left field, with no apparent context. He did like the medical school, but this seemed odd, to start the interview with a question like that. *Was this a test of some kind? A trick question? If he answered yes, would he seem to be sucking up? If he answered no, would he be labeled as a malcontent?* He decided not to over-analyze.

"Some days were hard, but most of the time I enjoyed the challenges," he ventured.

"What courses did you particularly like or dislike?"

"I guess Gross Anatomy was my least favorite. Memorizing all those body parts, the course of arteries, veins, and nerves, I wondered if I'd remember any of it. I took a surgery anatomy elective, though, in my junior year, and we dissected another cadaver. Surprisingly, a lot came back to me."

"And your favorite?"

"Community Pediatrics. Outpatient clinics. That seemed the most real to me of all the clinical rotations. I also loved my time on the pediatric wards here."

Ben paused, then asked, "May I ask what your field is, Dr. Caldwell?"

"Pediatric endocrinology. I'm particularly interested in growth hormone. Maybe I can get you interested," he chuckled.

"Well, I am interested in growth and development. Not necessarily the endocrine part of it, more the influence of a child's environment, family structure and dynamics."

"One of my colleagues, Dr. Frankel, runs a growth clinic that looks not only at hormonal influences but the impact of nutrition and social factors that affect growth," Caldwell said. "Fascinating confluence of factors there. She's published some landmark papers about that."

Their conversation spilled off in a lot of different directions and by the end of the half hour he had come to like Dr. Caldwell. When the pediatric resident, who was introduced to show him around, led him down the corridors, Ben realized he knew all about this hospital and although the resident was pleasant enough, Ben didn't relate to him the way he had related to Andrea Garrison at County.

He left Pediatric Children's with a visceral sense that he should train at Suffolk County Hospital. It fit the vision of his future perfectly. But how could he break this to his parents?

~~~

"How did the interviews go?" Jacob asked as soon as they came together for dinner that night.

"The interviews and the tours went very well at PCH and County," Ben answered cautiously, weighing his words carefully. "I liked them both."

"So, what do you think?" Jacob closed in.

"Well, first of all, Suffolk County Hospital's buildings aren't as bad as they look from the outside. And I could navigate the halls, the on-call rooms, the elevators, all those things looked good. Andrea, the resident who showed me around was great, happy to be there, a very warm person. The patients I saw had extremely interesting conditions. I liked it there."
~~~

"How did all that compare with Boston Pediatric?" Sophie said.

"My interview at Pediatric was also good. Course I know that hospital well, as a student and patient there. Guess who I saw just as I was getting on the elevator?"

"Dr. Weller?" Sophie asked.

"Nope. Cathy Kelly. You know, the nurse I told you about. The pretty one I met while I was in the hospital. Today she gave me her phone number. I'm to call her after dinner. Can't wait. She's special."

"Well, getting back to the issue of where to train," Jacob pressed on, ignoring Ben's mention of Cathy. "Have you formed any opinion?"

He took a deep breath, blew it all out, looked up at the ceiling, put his hands on the table.

"I liked Suffolk better. The whole package. I know you both want me to stay at Boston Pediatric, but remember, my advisor told me to carefully consider other places since I'd gone to Channing Medical School and Boston Pediatric is affiliated with Channing. He said I needed new perspective," Ben rattled on nervously. "And I saw this window into a different pediatric population at Suffolk and a different emphasis on mission. I think I like Suffolk better."

Ben stared at the dining room wallpaper, a floral pattern by Schumacher that Jacob had complained had cost too much. He waited for the expected eruption from his father and disapproval from his mother. Neither came.

"Your mother and I talked this over last night and we agreed this should be your decision. And it is. As you know, we preferred Boston Pediatric Hospital, but I can see you're more committed to the underserved population than I would be. Abraham's influence shows, and he's a good person to emulate."

Ben gave out a sigh of relief and smiled. He was also gratified that his father appreciated his brother after all those years of alienation.

"Thanks," was all he could say, as tears filled his eyes, and he considered how special his parents were.

"So, you better go call Cathy," Sophie said, smiling at her only child.

He wheeled into his room and groped through his pockets for Cathy's phone number. Where the hell did I put that paper? He finally found it in his pants pocket, laid it out on his desk, and with sweaty palms dialed the number.

"Hello."

"Hi, this is Ben. Cathy?"

"Oh, hi Ben," she sang. "Thanks for calling. Sorry I was abrupt today, but I had a doctor's appointment I had trouble getting, so I didn't want to cancel, even though I wanted to talk to you."

Tempted to ask what kind of doctor she was seeing and for what, he controlled his curiosity and said, "Would you like to have lunch or dinner sometime?"

"I'd love that. Have any favorite places?"

"Like Greek food?"

"Sure. Know a good place?"

"Where do you live?"

"Jamaica Plain."

"There's a good one on Route 9 in Chestnut Hill. That's easy for both of us. Called Christopher's. When are you free?"

"Saturdays are best for me. Let me look at my calendar."

Ben doodled on his note pad as his heart rate accelerated.

"How about next Saturday?"

"Great. Noon? Or six?"

"Noon's better. I have plans for later."

"Do you need a ride?"

"Let's just meet there. Got an address?"

Ben had been there many times. He told her the number and they were set.

Plans for later? What is that? Does she have a boyfriend? Well, course she does. A beautiful girl like that. I'm surprised she's not already married. During this post-World War II period, everyone seems to be getting married in their twenties.

He got there early, ensuring he could park and get into the restaurant without a struggle. He swiveled his legs sideways, grabbed his leg braces and fastened them onto his knees and followed what was now an established routine and then maneuvered his chair into the restaurant. He was breathing rapidly, recovering from an exertion known only to people with no function in their legs.

Ben sat in his wheelchair facing the entrance so he could watch for her. By the time she arrived a few minutes late, he'd already consumed two glasses of lemonade. He hoped he didn't have to go to the men's room.

"Ben, it's so good to see you. You look great! Let me hear all about you," Cathy said in her soothing alto voice.

"Um, well, I'm fine. And you look sensational. So glad to lay my eyes on you. Tell me what you're doing these days."

"No, no, you first. I can't wait another minute to find out what's going on with you."

Before he could begin, the waitress came and took their orders. It was a merciful break so he could collect his thoughts. He hated talking about his illness, his paralysis, and all that had transpired since he'd last seen this delightful girl. But he soldiered through talking about his experiences of the last few months.

When he was through, he looked at her damp eyes and knew he was falling in love. He feared this would happen, and he didn't want it to happen, for the outcome would most likely leave him depressed. It couldn't lead anywhere but to disappointment and still another loss.

He thought of Sandra. He hadn't heard from her since she came to visit. This relationship would probably follow that same trajectory.

Cathy reached over the table for Ben's hand as tears lined down her cheeks. "I promised myself I wouldn't do this, but here I am weeping. I'm sorry, but I feel for you so deeply. It must have been so awful for you. And you seem so strong despite it all. How do you do it?"

Ben repressed his own tears, glad to have the feel of her soft hands on his.

"How do I do it? Good question. Not alone. A whole lot of help. I've been blessed by the best parents ever, by friends, and colleagues, and countless people in the hospital and at Harley Rehab. I sure couldn't have done it by myself. I often think of patients who don't have any of the resources I've had. How do they cope? But somehow, many of them do, not only cope, but overcome odds I can't even imagine. Poverty. Bigotry. Violent homes. Limitations of all kinds. No one to advocate for them.

"But I also have moments where I don't feel so strong. All things considered, though, I'm doing reasonably well, better than I thought I would at first."

Their food arrived, breaking the somber mood. They both ate eagerly, glancing at one another, then smiles took over.

"Okay, it's your turn," Ben said. "Tell me everything," hoping she wouldn't tell him that she had this fantastic boyfriend.

"Well, I still work at Boston Pediatric, love my assignment these days in the postop surgery suite. I'm studying for my MPH at Channing School of Public Health. Won't finish that for a couple of years. Pretty boring life, actually. Live in Jamaica Plain in a cute little apartment above an Ethiopian restaurant. Great smells drift into my place. Walk around the Jamaica Pond at least four times a week."

Ben was hooked. He couldn't hesitate any longer.

"Do you have any special person?"

"Haven't had time. About the only boys I know now are medical people and they have no time either, so no, no special person." She cocked her head and looked directly at Ben. "Do you think something's wrong with me?"

"Are you kidding? You're, um, I don't know how to say this, so I'll just use the obvious words -- beautiful and nice. I'd take you out on a date in a New York minute."

There. He'd said it. Now what will be her reaction?

"Just ask."

Ben pressed his courage button and said, "Are you free tomorrow afternoon? It's Sunday and I'm free."

"Set a time," she said, smiling.

"Two?"

She told him her address and where he could park, "Not easy in JP, but I know some secret parking places."

She glided around the table, kissed him on the cheek, and bade him goodbye. Ben sat there, lovestruck, for the next ten minutes, then went back to his van and headed home, floating on a luxurious carpet of acceptance.

Chapter 18

Learning More

Saturday night, "the loneliest night of the week," and Ben was alone but far from lonely. The thought of his Sunday date with Cathy was tantalizing. He occupied himself, first by reading, which didn't work, then by listening to the Boston Celtics game with Sophie and Jacob, also avid fans.

This Celtics team was getting more interesting after a couple of losing seasons, now with the fiery and controversial Red Auerbach as their coach and Bob Cousy, the phenomenal but also controversial guard who'd played at Holy Cross. With Ed Macauley and Bill Sharman as able teammates, Cousy was tearing up the league. They'd lost the 1951 playoff game to the New York Knickerbockers, but this year, Cousy was averaging over 20 points per game. Tonight's game was no exception. Cousy scored 24 points and had 8 assists in his fast break style. Ben and his parents cheered them on in Ben's room.

Sunday's blazing sun rose over milky clouds and by afternoon was driving the winter temperature up to an unseasonable 45 degrees. The sky was translucent, its rays reflecting off Jamaica Pond, around which runners, dogwalkers, cyclists and roller skaters were moving on the well-kept pathways. The mood was celebratory after two weeks of gray wintry and frosty weather that had kept folks inside. Now there was liberty and freedom to enjoy the tease of Spring. In reality, sunny weather was still far away.

They had agreed to meet at the Pond rather than have Ben pick her up at her apartment. He parked the Suburban at a spot overlooking the Pond and waited in the car until he saw Cathy jogging over from her place. When she came to the driver's side, she said, "Let me cool down from my jog. If I don't, I'll cramp up a little." She did some stretching and then smiled at Ben.

"Ready now."

Since Cathy was there to help, he didn't need to go through his routine getting out of the car.

"I'll need your help getting my wheelchair from the back of the van," he said. "You'll see a pull cord for the ramp. Just pull it and the ramp will roll out onto the ground. Then you can push the wheelchair onto the ramp to get it down. Just bring it around to me and I'll show you my technique for getting out of the driver's seat and into the chair." He'd done this now so many times he was not self-conscious about it anymore.

"Let's go around the pond," Ben suggested after he was in his chair. They shared a hug, and she gave him a kiss on his cheek. "Just walk beside me. I can move the chair myself." He wanted to avoid any awkwardness and assure Cathy of his independent mobility.

They made small talk as they moved around the pond, avoiding dogwalkers and joggers. Coming back to their starting point Cathy said, "I can fix lunch at my place if you'd like."

"Sounds great to me. You can also show me this secret parking place you told me about."

He described his routine for getting back into the driver's seat while he pulled on the grab bar and lifted himself into position behind the wheel. She got the chair back into the rear of the van, reversing the procedure she'd used in getting it out. She was a quick learner. Once she was seated in the passenger side, Ben showed her the clever accelerator and brake controls that allowed him to drive.

"Wow, that's amazing. I wondered how you were able to drive. I'm impressed." What she didn't say was that she was relieved and reassured since he was going to drive her home.

Once in her kitchen, Ben was able to relax after being hoisted up the stairs by two strong young men, waiters from the Ethiopian restaurant downstairs who had seen them coming. He was no longer embarrassed by his inability to perform such everyday tasks, having come to terms with his limitations and constantly telling himself to accentuate the positives in his life.

Cathy got busy putting together sandwiches and salad for their lunch. Ben was taking in her small apartment and all the personal things that spoke of her interests and preferences for color, style, and tastes. Her favorite colors were strong greens, blues, and reds. She had some original art, watercolors mainly, but a few sculptures, and wood carvings of birds and other small animals. Two small Oriental prayer rugs were in her living room, with an antique love seat in brocaded fabric and a leather recliner chair. Her bookcases were cinder blocks and boards overflowing with a jumble of books. He loved seeing her apartment, the little touches that helped define this young woman who was becoming so dear to him.

They sat at a modest maple dropleaf table by one of the two windows in her tiny apartment, facing Center Street with its trolley tracks and pedestrians. Ben couldn't stop looking at Cathy as she ate. Their conversation was stilted at first, but then they both relaxed and laughed about their experiences in the hospital. Turning more serious, Ben was eager to learn more about Cathy. He hardly knew her, and she knew even less about him. They were both nervous and this, their "first date," led to the usual questions about where they'd grown up, their school experiences -- all the getting-to-know-you inquiries. Ben quickly told her a little about his parents, his home in Chestnut Hill, his college days, and Channing Medical School. Then he wanted to know about her.

"Well, as you can tell from my name, I'm of Irish descent. Grew up in South Boston, have three brothers and one sister. I'm the youngest, so I'm spoiled, according to my siblings. I went to Catholic school, and then to Villanova for my bachelor's in science in nursing. You probably know the nurse's dorm across from the Fenway Building. That's where I lived for three years while I got my master's in nursing. Easy to cross the street to do my training.

"My parents are still living where they've always lived, on D Street in Southie. My older brothers are all married and raising families. My sister and I are spinsters." They both laughed at the term.

"So, what are your plans for the future?"

"Unclear. I like bedside nursing for now, but that's hard to do as one gets older. I'm thinking of getting a second master's, in public health or something along administrative lines. What're you going to do?"

"Just decided I want to go to Suffolk County Hospital for my residency in pediatrics. I think I'd like to teach. And see patients. I'm also interested in public health. As you know, being wheelchair-bound makes choices a little narrower, but I've learned to do most things I used to do. Course, I can't ride a bike, play baseball, hike, and stuff like that. But I can still swim. Remember FDR? He did a lot of swimming. Strengthens your upper body and your lungs and heart get a good workout by swimming laps."

"I admire your courage. I remember seeing you in the hospital. It must've been hard."

"It was, but that's past. You probably saw me at my lowest point. But I've had so much help and encouragement—from my parents, colleagues, faculty, and friends. And my Uncle Abraham. He died recently, but he was an inspiration in all kinds of ways. I'll tell you about him sometime. What do you do for fun? Hobbies, sports, movies, books?"

Ben couldn't get enough information about Cathy.

"Love fiction, especially romantic fiction. I like some mysteries, mostly Agatha Christie. Since I don't like violence in any form, cozy mysteries are better for me. I like historical biographies too. As far as sports are concerned, I don't like football, but I love baseball and basketball."

Ben's eye lit up. "My two sports too! We have to take in some Red Sox games this summer. And the Celtics play in the Garden next week. Wanna go?"

"Love to. When?"

"I'll find out and let you know.'

Ben didn't want this day to end, but he also didn't want to appear to be hogging her time. He could stay with her for hours, but he thought he'd better be discreet and end on a good note.

"Can you see me out? And call your buddies downstairs to help me downstairs? I hope they're always available when I visit you."

"There's always someone downstairs at the restaurant ready to help. They're wonderful people. I'll call them."

On his way home, Ben was aware they hadn't touched on some important and obvious challenges: *Where could this relationship possibly go? I'm not an ordinary person. I'm disabled, no way to put a pretty face on that. I'm Jewish, she's Catholic. Opposite poles. What would Sophie and Jacob think of his dating a "shicksa?" What would her parents think of her dating, not only a paralyzed man, but a Jew?*

Chapter 19

Family Meeting

Events overtook Ben during the next week. Acceptance letters arrived from both Boston Pediatric Hospital and Suffolk County Hospital. His medical school record, his faculty recommendations and his interviews apparently overshadowed any concerns by the respective Residency Committees about Ben's paralysis. As the lone female member of the Suffolk County Residency Committee said during the intern ranking session, "Accepting Ben Levinson is a strong statement of this institution's commitment to leading the way for inclusion of a different kind of candidate in this cadre of young doctors. The next step will be to equalize the acceptance of women and minorities into our program."

Ben received both letters on the same day after a stressful day in his surgery rotation. A day like this made it clear that surgery was not for him, not only because of the physical demands of long hours in the operating room. Most important, he saw that spending this amount of time with a single anesthetized patient was not how he wanted to practice medicine. He was more attuned to relating to patients while they were conscious and responsive, spending time talking and listening to them.

He saved the news of his acceptance letters until dinner with his parents, a time traditionally reserved for talking about what mattered to each of them, what went on in their lives that day, and general news of the day. He'd always looked forward to dinner for this intimate sharing, and tonight would be one of the more exciting ones. The acceptance letters would take top billing, but he also wanted to tell them about Cathy. He was anxious about both. He couldn't be sure of his parents' reception to either item. But even so, he could hardly wait.

"I ran into Deb Robbins at the Stop and Shop this morning," Sophie said, once everyone was served. "She told me that her son, Josh -- do you know him, Ben?"

"I knew he was in our class. He was very quiet. Nice enough, but we never really connected."

"Well, he just got accepted into the Wharton Business School in Philly."

"Not surprising. He seemed sort of like an accountant," Ben said, showing little interest in this news, anxious to talk about his own. He hurried things along by asking, "Anything new downtown, Dad?"

"Yeah, for some reason, we had a record day for engagement rings," Jacob said. "Don't know why.

Funny time of the year for it. Usually happens in the Spring."

It was finally Ben's turn.

"Got some interesting mail today," he said, teasing his parents' curious natures.

"And?" Sophie said, taking the bait.

"Acceptances from both hospitals."

"That's great news!" Jacob exclaimed and Sophie cried "Hooray! Wonderful!" After a pause, Jacob said, "Did getting accepted at Boston Pediatric alter your decision to go to County?"

Sophie and Jacob's eyes fixed on Ben. His gaze darted back and forth from one to the other as he considered his answer.

"I was flattered to get both letters," he said. "Very affirming for my feeling of self-worth. I'll always treasure this day as the true beginning of my medical career."

"Are you being deliberately coy in answering my question?" Jacob said. Ben thought this was a rather rude way of forcing him to answer, but he repressed his feelings and forged ahead anyhow.

"No, my decision is Suffolk County Hospital. I simply feel it's the right decision for me and one I'm very comfortable with."

Jacob looked down at his plate, dabbed his napkin on his lips, and said, "I sincerely hope you don't regret that decision. This really sets the rudder for your career. What do you think, Sophie?"

Turning to Ben and taking his hand, Sophie said, "Well, as you probably have figured out, we hoped you would take Boston Pediatric if you were accepted. We thought maybe you'd settled on County because you doubted you'd get in at Boston Pediatric. So, now, since you could take your training at Boston Pediatric, I think both of us are somewhat disappointed. But if County is where you want to go, we'll be rooting for your success there." A squeeze of her hand was reassuring.

Is this the time to bring up Cathy? Ben wondered. Might as well get it out there. It's not a fait accompli anyhow, it's a work in progress.

"There's another thing I want to discuss with you," looking again back and forth between the two most important people in his life. "You knew I spent Sunday afternoon with my friend Cathy Kelly. It was very pleasant, and frankly, I'm very fond of her. Our relationship is in the very earliest of stages, so nothing can be predicted. But I really like her, and I think she likes me. We're going to continue to see each other and see what may come to pass."

"Her surname is Kelly?" Jacob said. "I assume she's Irish. And Catholic?"

"Yes, and yes." He didn't ask if he had a problem with that. He didn't need to.

"Wasn't she the nurse you knew from the hospital? She saw you once in your room at the hospital?" Sophie asked.

"Yes, she still works at Boston Pediatric for now. She got her nursing degree from Villanova, and now is considering getting a master's degree in public health from Channing."

"Know anything about her family?" Jacob asked.

"Only what she told me: three brothers, one sister, all adults and on their own. She's the baby of the family. Her parents still live in South Boston."

"Do you have any idea how she feels about your paralysis?" Jacob asked Ben the obvious question.

"She's always been sympathetic. But if you mean, how does she feel about getting involved with a guy who's paralyzed, I have no way of knowing. She seems to accept me as I am, but, as I said before, it's early. This will have to be addressed, depending on how this plays out, in due time."

"She's aware you're Jewish?" Sophie said.

"With a name like Levinson, it's pretty apparent."

"What do you suppose her folks will think if this goes beyond a friendship?"

"No idea. Hasn't come up."

"Well, as you say, this is early, and so we'll just have to see," Sophie said.

Jacob moved his chair away from the table and stood up. "I agree. We'll just wait and see where this goes.

"Wow, this has been quite a load of news. Ben, can we have a private conversation?" Jacob asked.

"Sure. Here, or in my room?"

"Let's go to your room."

"I'll clean up," Sophie said, rising from the table and beginning to collect dirty dishes. "Let me know when you two are finished."

The two men moved to Ben's room, closed the door. Jacob sat on the love seat, Ben sitting opposite him in his wheelchair.

"You may know what I'm going to say," Jacob said.

"You are wondering if I can perform sexually," Ben said, unblinking. "That's why we're in here without Mom."

"Right. I haven't had the nerve to talk with you about this before, but now it's acutely important with this new romantic interest in your life. Seems I should discuss it with you. Hope you don't feel this violates your privacy."

"No, I'm glad to talk about it. Um, the question is: Can I get an erection, right?"

"Right." Jacob was surprised and pleased that Ben was so forthright.

"The answer is yes. The first time I was sure of it was when Sandra -- you remember her, don't you? She was here recently, you were at work, and she kissed me a long time, on the lips, and I got an erection. I have since had several, especially when I first wake up in the morning."

"Well, congratulations!" Jacob laughed and Ben joined him with a chuckle.

"So that's really the only thing I wanted to talk to you about man to man. I thought it might embarrass Sophie – and you -- to bring it up in front of her. The other things about this new relationship, the differences between you two, the religious things, the family things, these can all wait until we know where this is going. No point in getting all worried about something that might never happen."

He thinks, maybe hopes, this will fizzle out. I suppose it could. But he's right, only time will tell. I'd sure love to know what his private thoughts are about this, and Sophie's too.

Jacob got up, gave Ben a pat on the shoulder, went to the door and called Sophie to come into Ben's room.

"Our private conversation is over. Dishes all set?"

The Levinson's spent the rest of the evening reading and listening to music, their way of relaxing after this dinner of revelations.

Chapter 20

Getting to Know You

Ben lost no time responding to Boston Pediatric and Suffolk County Hospitals. He awoke around 5AM and wrote two letters, politely thanking and saying no to the former and yes to Suffolk County's offer. He did this with a new certainty of purpose. He didn't second guess himself, gaining a surer confidence in having considered all the elements of his decision. This was his preferred path forward, one he'd carefully and deliberately chosen and would live with, whatever the consequences. Once he'd put these letters in the mail, he felt a new lightness of being and a freedom he hadn't felt since polio struck him. It had been a hard six months.

He rolled into the surgical ward for rounds a little early, even for surgeons, who make rounds before operating, so they were famously early birds. He greeted his fellow students as they came.

"Alex, Steve, Margaret. Have you heard back about your internships?"

"Got mine from U of Chicago," Steve said. "Real happy I got in there. Hard one to get."

"Rotating or straight?" Ben asked.

"Rotating. Straights are more competitive, and anyway, I wanted general grounding before I decide on a specialty. I'm not even sure what I want to do. I may go into general practice."

The others all got their choices, not unusual for graduates of Channing. No one else was staying in Boston, underscoring Ben's advisor's suggestion to go elsewhere for training.

After the day's grueling surgery schedule, Ben went home and called Cathy.

"Hi. Ben here. How're you doin'?"

"Doing well, you?"

"Good." A deep breath. "Want to get together again?"

"Yes, I'd like that. When?"

"Are you free this weekend?"

After comparing calendars, they decided on Saturday evening at the Ethiopian restaurant downstairs from Cathy's apartment. When Saturday afternoon arrived, Ben paced around his room, fidgeted with his shirt, wondering if he should wear a tie or not. He decided not, but then, what about a sports coat? He forced himself to calm down, impatiently awaiting the appointed time.

He went early because he had a lot to do just to get out of his car and into the restaurant. Once he parked in the secret place Cathy had told him about, he went into his routine for getting into his wheelchair, then maneuvered his chair into the restaurant. He was breathing rapidly, recovering from an exertion known only to people with no function in their legs.

Cathy was already there, talking to two waitresses when Ben arrived. She waved and hurried over to meet him at the door.

"Right on time. Is that something you always do, get to places on time?"

"Pretty much. Especially when it's to meet you," he said, hearing giggles from the two waitresses, who then left them alone.

"What should I order? You probably eat here often, right?" Ben said.

She pointed to several items on the menu and one of the waitresses came back and took their orders. Other hungry patrons came in and slowly the other seven tables filled up in this small, intimate eatery. When their dinners came, they both began eating with gusto. As their early hunger was sated and their pace slowed, Ben ventured into bland conversation, stumbling over his words at first, but soon he found his footing.

"What was your week like?"

"Nothing special. Yours?"

Leaning forward, hands animatedly accenting his words, Ben told her about his acceptance letters and the discussion with his parents.

"Boy, compared to my boring week, yours was full of action! Didn't you tell me your parents wanted you to stay at Pediatric Hospital?"

"Yeah, they worried about County, the neighborhood, what they'd read and heard about the chaos there. The conversation was a little stressful, honestly. But my parents are the best. They're very supportive of my decisions—always have been. You'll have to meet them sometime."

He immediately regretted saying this, knowing how presumptuous it was suggesting the "meet the parents" should happen so soon in their budding relationship. But she greeted this casually.

"I'd love meeting them. They sound so lovable."

"Really? I worried you'd think meeting my parents was premature."

"It's not as though this means anything nowadays," Cathy said. "Life is pretty informal now. You know, peace and prosperity, and all that Eisenhower rhetoric. Actually, it's not so much his rhetoric as that of his advisors."

Ben has always paid a lot of attention to national politics. He was trying to adapt to this new president, whose early actions seemed, so far, quite innocuous. Since she mentioned Eisenhower, he was curious about her political orientation and wondered if he should ask her about it. Uncertain about discussing this with a woman he hardly knew, he went ahead and asked anyway. *Why not?*

"Speaking of Eisenhower, what flavor of politics do you like?"

"I'm a lifelong Democrat, just like my parents. Not a marcher, or political junkie or anything like that, but I tend to be liberal. My Democratic Party is a little different, I think, from my parent's Democratic Party."

Ben let out a long breath, smiled and said,

"Me too. Not sure what you mean about your Democratic Party not being your parents.' In Boston I think most people are Democrats, right?"

"Democrats, yes, but not necessarily liberal. That's what I meant. I grew up in South Boston. A lot of bigotry there. You'd think Irish people would be tolerant of minorities since the Irish were discriminated against early on, you know, the Help Wanted signs in businesses that said: "No Irish Need Apply" or simply "NINA" which was understood by the Irish. But there is such tribalism in Irish communities, and they -- we -- are so thoroughly indoctrinated Catholics, some of us have a hard time seeing others' opinions."

Ben had no idea he would open such a Pandora's jar of feelings. But he loved it. And her, for rebelling against the things in her upbringing she didn't agree with.

"You know I'm Jewish, right? I'm one of those minorities who feel discriminated against."

"Of course, I know you're Jewish," she laughed. "But I'm kind of a rebel, you know. And I'm curiously attracted to people different from the ones I grew up with, all of them so predictable and too much alike. You're interesting in all kinds of ways," she smiled.

Ben grinned back, not sure in what way he was "interesting." Was it because he was Jewish, or because he was disabled? Or for other reasons? In any event, he was flattered that she thought him so.

"I told my parents about you," he said. "They wondered what your parents would think when you told them you're seeing a Jewish boy."

"They probably wouldn't like it much. But I don't really know since I've never dated anyone outside of the 'tribe' before."

"I bet you've been popular, within the 'tribe,'" Ben said, eager to know more about her romantic past.

"Yeah, like most of my girlfriends, I've had lots of dates, I've kissed a lot of frogs hoping they'd turn into princes, but none ever did. Never had anyone I'd jump off a cliff for. And as for my parents, they know me and know they better not interfere in my choices. They know I have very strong convictions. And they know they can't dictate to me."

Wow. She's one high-spirited woman. As I get to know her better, I like her -- dare I say love her? -- even more. But aside from our differing backgrounds, we haven't talked about a multitude of things that affect people's relationships, like the biggie -- my paralysis -- at all. Never been mentioned. I don't know or have the faintest notion about how to broach that subject. Maybe head-on?

But before Ben could raise this, she said, with a smile, "So, what do your parents think about your seeing an Irish Catholic lass?"

"Good question. I have an idea, but they haven't said anything. You know what some Jews would call you?"

"Shicksa," she quickly retorted. "A term well-known to us potential shicksas. I also know what that entails for us as non-Jews. Rejection. Cast out. Makes one think twice."

"And that's still not a non-starter?"

"No. You know, personal relationships depend on individuals, not groups. From what you've told me about them, I would guess your parents are comfortable with 1950's realities, which to me seem a lot different than they were just a few years ago. But I also am aware I'm looking at the world with twenty-four-year-old eyes."

"Hard to say what my folks think. They're circumspect about a lot of things. They're traditionalists, not surprising given their history. They left Germany at the early years of fascism and although they don't ever speak about it, it's ingrained in their psyches. And they are avid readers of news.

"I don't think I've ever told you about my Uncle Abraham. He got out in the nick of time, in 1939, but he lived through horrific times before he got out. When he came here, my parents took him in without a second thought. He became a second father to me, a role model in so many ways."

Ben began to choke up, recalling Abraham, and how much he meant to him. He stopped talking, took a few deep breaths. Cathy reached over and took his hand. He recovered his composure, put his hand over Cathy's and was able to continue.

"You mentioned tribalism when you described your South Boston neighborhood. Jews are that way too. Maybe even stronger because of anti-Semitism, both overt and covert."

"When you describe your Uncle Abraham, you speak of him in the past tense," Cathy said.

"He died not too long ago. I miss him every day."

"I'm sorry. I wish I'd known him, especially since he meant so much to you. You'll have to tell me more about him."

Ben looked at Cathy and realized something special was going on. He felt weightless. He saw tears in her eyes, and he wanted to hold her so they could share this moment. What could he do? He could only wait for her to come around the table to him. Only then did he gaze around the restaurant to see that it had emptied out and they were the only diners left.

"I'm amazed. We're keeping the waitresses late. It shows how talkative I am when I have a good listener. Good thing you don't have far to go home."

"I'm a good listener to someone who has such interesting things to say. I'm glad you've told me about your family, and your uncle. It makes me understand you better."

"Now you need to tell me more about you," Ben said, thinking he'd monopolized the conversation.

"Come upstairs if you'd like, and I can tell you more about myself," she said.

"I'll need help getting upstairs. Then there's the problem of getting back down and to my car."

"I'll ask the guys to help you upstairs. You can call your folks from my apartment and tell them you'll see them tomorrow."

Chapter 21

Even More

It snowed during the night. When Ben woke up, he looked out over Center Street and was surprised to see snowplows clearing the street. Trolleys not running. The world was serene, the usual bustle silenced by Sunday lethargy and weather conditions. In these unfamiliar surroundings, he was blissfully happy. Cathy was in her kitchen and the aroma of Arabica coffee suffused the apartment.

"You awake?" she called as she heard stirrings from the bedroom.

"Yup. How long you been up?"

"Not long. Like breakfast?"

"Hungry as a horse. But I'd rather have you back here in bed. After I grope my way to the bathroom."

"Need help? I think your crutches are right by the bed."

Ben went to the bathroom on his crutches, then eased himself into his wheelchair. As he entered the kitchen he saw Cathy, still in her nightgown. She treaded silently to his side, kissing him as she caressed his neck.

"What did your parents say when you told them you were going to spend the night with an Irish lassie?"

Laughing, he said, "they wished me good luck."

"I think I'll like your parents! Well, you didn't need good luck. You were wonderful."

Ben's performance anxiety had been painfully intense. This was the first time since he was paralyzed that he had attempted to make love. Ben, trying to get into what he considered the customary male dominant position on top of Cathy, was grabbing the sides of the bed to pull himself into position, with his flaccid legs pinning down Cathy's legs. They finally looked at each other and began giggling at the absurdity of their situation. When the spasms of laughter subsided, it was clear that Cathy knew intuitively how to proceed with Ben's limitations of motion. She lovingly persuaded him to lie on his back and she did the rest. If Ben had any doubt about his feelings for Cathy, they completely fell away. He felt his life taking on a completely new arc.

"So, you said you were hungry," Cathy said. "I can offer scrambled eggs, kiwi fruit, sourdough toast, jam, orange or cranberry juice, and coffee, all available. What's your pleasure?"

"Well, I'll take all those things. Where do you want me?"

"Right where you are. I have this serving tray that will fit nicely across your wheelchair arms."

After they both ate and went back to bed for another session of lovemaking and slumber, they began conversation anew.

"Have you thought about the implications of a relationship with a paraplegic?" Ben said, finally screwing up his courage to discuss this.

"Of course. Haven't ignored the obvious. You may wonder about my sort of laidback attitude toward this. To help explain it, let me tell you about my Aunt Tess, my mother's sister. She lived down the street from us," Cathy said.

"Tess -- we all called her Tess though her name was Theresa -- was a nurse, worked in the ER at Carney Hospital. I adored her. She was someone I wanted to be. An inveterate athlete, she loved hiking, running, playing field hockey, but closest to her heart was horseback riding. She owned a beautiful chestnut mare named Fawn, kept her in a stable on the South Shore.

"One day she was out riding Fawn in a wooded area near the stable. She told me she was distracted by a deer in a copse of trees when Fawn ran under a tree with a low-hanging branch. Tess didn't see it until it was too late. The branch caught her in the neck, catapulted her to the ground. She struggled to get onto her feet. Fawn came back, her nose nuzzling Tess. But she couldn't move her legs. Another rider saw her down, came over to check on her, and after seeing her plight, told her she'd get help and rode quickly back to the stable and called an ambulance.

"The ambulance was there within minutes, the attendants gently lifting her onto a firm board and stabilizing her neck before speeding off to the hospital.

"At the hospital X-rays showed multiple fractured thoracic vertebrae. They took her to the operating room, but her thoracic spine was shattered in so many places, the surgeons couldn't fix it.

"I was ten years old. I spent a lot of time with her during her rehab and my respect and admiration for her grew and grew. She took on her disability with a vengeance, eventually was able to return to nursing as an administrator with the local Visiting Nurses Association.

"So, I have some experience with this. I see it in a different way from most people. I recognize courage and I'm a little blind to the inability to do things."

"She must be a tough cookie. Quite a story. I assume she's retired now like your mom. If possible, I'd like to meet her and get her advice on coping," Ben said.

"Here's my take on things," he continued. "I've come to somewhat of an accommodation with this. It's taken time, but now I'm determined to do everything I'm capable of, adjust to my life as I find it. I intend to live to the max. I want a family, want to be a good husband and father. I want to teach and practice general pediatrics, do what I can with people with disabilities, both physical and mental. I want to influence neophyte doctors, nurses, and social workers to be the best they can be, not only as professional health care providers, but as full human beings. I want to improve health care for poor people, like my uncle did. Those are my goals."

Cathy was lying on her side, facing Ben as she listened to this man with whom she had just spent a wonderful night. When he stopped talking, she rolled closer, gave him a lingering kiss.

"Since I first saw you when you were a patient in the hospital, I've thought of you every day," she said. "But I admired you before that day, from afar, and after we met that day, I began caring deeply for you. I've never felt this way before about a man, and don't know where this feeling comes from, but I'm not trying to figure it out. It's just there.

"That's my story and I'm sticking to it," she laughed.

Ben couldn't believe his good fortune in meeting this remarkable woman. How did it happen? What gods brought this person into his life? A most unlikely matching, if one dissected it, but, upon further inspection, they were alike in the ways that mattered. Both health care providers, caretakers of people, empathic in their relationships, optimistic idealists, and young enough to have not developed cynicism.

"It's time to hear your story," Ben said, a little apprehensive as he gazed at the woman with whom he was beginning to anticipate a lifetime together.

"Um, where to begin. Well, for starters, I'm something of a tomboy. Considering I have three older brothers, not surprising. Being the youngest, I also was a bit of a curiosity to them, even though they had another older sister. My brothers were good to me, letting me tag along with them to their baseball, basketball, and football practices. That's what got me interested in sports. I learned not to care for football, though, when I was a student nurse. Saw too many head and back injuries.

"Childhood was classic South Boston, typical Catholic schools with nuns, some good, some awful, and the whole nine yards of Catholic brainwashing. I was one of the good girls, though."

"Were there any colored people in South Boston?"

"You must be kidding. No. No Jews either. We had some Italian families, but predominantly Irish. Ward-healers lived in our neighborhood."

"Ward-healers?"

"The ward part referred to the voting ward. You needed something; you knew who to call. I guess that's why they were called 'healers.' Very tight.

"A lot of alcohol and frequent fights among the young guys. My brothers were pugnacious, but when the fights were over, the kids made up. Don't know why that happened. Reminded me of a litter of puppies fighting, and then playing with each other. But boy, don't let somebody out of Southie try to take advantage of any of the guys in the neighborhood. Talk about tribalism."

"Did you go to high school there too?"

"Yeah, no discussion about that. Parochial school was the only choice, according to my parents, and they somehow raised the money for tuition, and I went. I was an honor roll student—pardon the self-congratulation—and I got a full scholarship to Villanova."

"That the first time you were out of South Boston?"

"Very first time, really. My family never went on trips or vacations. Couldn't afford them. We had good ole Carson Beach and spent our summers swimming there. Great memories. So, going away from Boston to college was a wild ride for me. Still a Catholic school, Villanova has a beautiful campus and a great place to get my BSN."

Ben couldn't help wondering about her boyfriends, this vast army of fantasy guys he was so jealous of. She had to have had them, as attractive and wonderful as she was. But he couldn't bring himself to ask, and in truth, he didn't really want to hear about them. But he was still curious.

"So, after Villanova you came back to Boston and went to work at Pediatric?"

"Yeah, but I worked first at Carney, just like Tess, for a few months before the job opened at Pediatric. I was lucky to get that job at such a prestigious place. And it opened up a world where not everyone was Catholic."

"If you get a slot at Channing Public Health School, when would that start?"

"Fall 1953. Wish me luck."

"You'll get in, I know it," he said, his affection for her taking precedence over clear-headed calculation. "How long will that take?"

"Two years minimum. Depends on whether I specialize in something."

He hesitated before asking, "Is it expensive?"

"Yeah, but I've been saving, and I'd get some financial aid."

"So, you and I will be in our training programs over the next two or three years. I'll be busy as hell, on duty every other night for the first year. Your schedule won't be that demanding. We need to figure out how to spend the little free time we'll have together," Ben said.

Am I being ridiculously presumptuous? After one night together? Does she see the same future as I? But I can't stand the thought of being without her. Is this because I'm so relieved that anyone will accept me as I am?

"We can work that out," Cathy said as she rolled away from Ben and stood up, stretching her arms over her head with a big yawn. "Internships are a punishment for all your sins, you know," she laughed.

"I think medical schools and hospitals are run by a sadistic group of aging men."

"And we accept it as though it's the only way we can become real doctors, Ben said. "It's absurd, the way we accept such things, as though it's the rites of initiation for the fraternity of Aesculapius. But 'twas ever thus. I just hope I can get through it okay."

Chapter 22

Adam Fisher, Summer 1953

Weekends together came to a sudden and inevitable end when Ben's internship began. He and Cathy were on the phones daily, but their in-person intimate romantic liaisons were on hold, at least for the present.

"Your description of sadistic old men running training programs was apt," Ben told Cathy after a grueling week of sleep deprivation. They were together for a short time on Sunday afternoon. "I'm seeing fascinating cases, but I'm wiped out all the time. I thought my effort just getting around was the reason, but everybody says they're exhausted."

"We have to be philosophical about this year. Next year, hopefully, won't be as bad," Cathy said.

"Have you heard from Channing yet?" Ben asked.

"Expect to this week. Wish me luck."

She took his hand and said, "Any time we can be together? Even just for lunch or dinner? I miss you so much."

"I miss you too. I go off oncology end of the month. Next month is outpatient and emergency room, should be a little lighter. Still have night call, but maybe we can squeeze in a couple of times together. We knew it was gonna be this way. Still not as bad as being a patient. I'll never forget that."

~~~

"Dr. Levinson, come to the Emergency Room STAT, the nurse said over the phone.

Ben had gone to bed around eleven and had just gotten to sleep when this call came. He was now accustomed to a routine when getting out of bed and into his wheelchair with a minimum of moves. He sped out of the on-call room and fidgeted with his scrub suit ties, cinching them up as he waited for the elevator. When the doors slid open, he wheeled across the narrow gap, swung the chair around, punched "B." When he arrived at the basement level, he raced his chair down the corridor to the ER.

"Hi Ben, good you're here," the nurse said briskly, "we have this four-year-old girl, Molly's her name, with long-lasting seizures, shipped in from St. Elsewhere. They tried everything there, but she keeps on convulsing. She needs a cut-down for an IV infusion. She's got tiny veins, nobody can find one, let alone get a needle in. Someone said you're good at doing cutdowns, so get on into Room 3 and do your thing. Susan's already setting up in there."
~~~

Ben had developed a sure-fire technique for cut downs, a procedure involving making an incision over the site of a vein. He was able to get this one done in jig-time. As soon as the needle was in, the anti-convulsant medication was infused. Molly's seizure gradually diminished, then stopped altogether. Ben looked at Susan and they both smiled at their success. Ben went out to the waiting room and found Molly's parents who were pacing around the small waiting room, mother crying and father trying to comfort her while he himself was trembling with fear. They looked at Ben quizzically. A doctor in a wheelchair?

"Good news, folks," Ben said. He saw their skepticism about his being in a wheelchair, decided not to address it. "Seizures have stopped. Molly's looking a whole lot better. Go in and give her a big hug." Mother sobbed even louder, but now they were signs of relief, not sorrow.

Ben looked at his watch, 2:20 AM. He wondered if he could get enough sleep not to be a zombie on rounds at 8. He turned around in his chair and was headed to the elevator when a nurse caught up with him.

"Sorry, but another case is on the way in from the Cape. Near-drowning. Eight-year-old boy. Tide pulled him out last evening on one of the beaches. Stabilized in a Cape hospital, be here in ten minutes. Prognosis poor."

"Any other history? Resuscitation measures? Has he vomited? Vitals in the ambulance?"

"He did vomit, but in these cases, there's always a question of aspiration. His oxygen sat no good. Blue fingers and toes. BP 90/50. Heart rate 110. Lungs full of noise, according to the ambulance guys."

Ben looked up non-fatal immersion in his handbook, known colloquially by the house staff as their "peripheral brains." When the ambulance arrived, the personnel handed him the records from the outside hospital. There were good notations that included the duration of the submersion and the time of the first breath after resuscitation. When they arrived, they hustled the kiddo into the ER and Ben took one look at him and said, "Get arterial blood gases stat. CBC and lytes. Ditto portable chest x-rays. Put in a bladder cath, monitor all intake and output of fluids. Check the airway and clear if not already clear. Positive pressure oxygen administration," Ben reeling off the orders. "Call ICU to tell them we're going to send this little guy up as soon as possible. What's his name?"

"Danny McCord. His parents are coming by their own car and will be here shortly. The ambulance attendants want to know if they can leave."

"I think so. I need to speak to them before they go," Ben said. He wheeled out to the ambulance where the driver was standing. "Good job, fellas. He's in good hands now, going to the ICU. Thanks for your help."

Turning to one of the nurses, he said, "Let me know when Danny's parents get here so I can talk to them. I'm sure they're beside themselves with worry. Can you imagine what it must be like to have your precious kid be so close to death? I can't conceive of it. I have no children myself, so it's unknown territory for me personally."

"I have a boy about that age," one of the nurses said. "I can tell you, it's scary all the things that can go wrong, even when you do everything you're supposed to. I bet Danny's parents are feeling guilty. I pray this kid pulls through."

Danny had not been in good shape when he arrived, but the crack team in the ER stabilized him and sent him quickly to the Pediatric ICU. Ben intercepted Danny's parents and reassured them that Danny was stable and that he was going to the PICU.

"We should never have allowed him to go back into the water, but he said he wanted to take a quick swim before we went home. He's a strong swimmer for an eight-year-old and very head-strong. But we should have said no," his mother lamented to Ben.

"Not your fault. How could you have known there was a strong undertow? You couldn't. This was a freak accident. Don't blame yourselves. You pulled him out in time. Leave the rest up to us. We'll do our best."

He sent them to the PICU and hoped Danny would be okay. But he was worried and wondered if he'd overpromised.

It was almost five o'clock. Ben was deliberating whether he should go back to the on-call room or hit the cafeteria for some breakfast. His stomach answered the question, so he headed to the all- night cafeteria. This place was always busy, even at this hour.

He filled his tray with bacon, eggs, toast, orange juice and a big cup of coffee and headed toward a place where he could move his chair beside the table. Luckily the table was high enough for the arms of his chair to slip under. He avoided one corner of the dining area where smoking was allowed.

His history of asthma had made the decision for him never to smoke and he couldn't tolerate even being close to cigarette smoke. He couldn't understand why people smoked anyway. One of his professors--a surgeon—gave a lecture one day showing the lung tumors. He told the class to stop smoking because he claimed smoking caused lung cancer. Some students stopped, but many were skeptical and continued, since the ads for cigarettes featured men in white coats—supposed to be doctors—advocating smoking.

Ben felt almost normal after quaffing down his breakfast. He knew a long day awaited him. Maybe he could take a quickie nap before rounds. He went to the on-call room, lay down on the bed and was asleep in minutes. One of his roommates soon woke him for rounds.

~~~
~~~

Awake, Ben hurried off to morning rounds, the term given to the exercise of going around the ward to see all the patients.

"Dr. Levinson, you were in the ER when the near drowning came in. You want to fill us in?" Dr. Howard, their preceptor, said.

"You mean Danny?" Ben said, consistently referring to his patients with their names. He told Danny's story to the group, although he didn't know what had happened during the several hours since he admitted him.

"Well, Danny's sitting up in his bed, eating his breakfast. You must have magical powers," Dr. Howard laughed. "In future, we'll assign you to all near drownings."

Ben smiled with satisfaction, not because he thought he could take any credit for Danny's recovery, but simply happy this kid had gotten so much better.

After rounds, Ben spent the next several hours checking on his other patients, making progress notes and attending to all the scut work interns must do. He finished around one o'clock and went for lunch.

"Mind if I join you?" Adam Fisher asked. Ben recognized him from the early meetings all the interns had but hadn't really gotten to know him since he was on other rotations. He was easy to spot, being very large muscular colored man with bushy hair and an easy smile.

"Sure, have a seat. Glad to have company."

"Where you from?" Adam said.

"I'm a local boy. Born and bred in Boston. You?"

"Cambridge, but not Massachusetts. The town I come from is in Maryland, eastern shore of Chesapeake Bay. Can't seem to leave the east coast."

"You go to Hopkins?"

"University of Maryland. That other school in Baltimore."

"Is Suffolk County comparable to where you went?"

"Very much like Baltimore City Hospital. I'm attracted to inner city medicine. Maybe because I'm the color I am. Where did you go to Medical School?"

"Channing."

"Couldn't you get into Boston Pediatric?"

Boy, he's really direct.

"I got in but chose to come here. One of my advisors told me to spread my wings and get a different perspective."

"It's early, but you happy here?"

"Very. My advisor was right. I never saw anything like these cases at Boston Pediatric."

Adam, restless in his seat, looked intently at Ben across the table. He finally said, "Why the wheelchair?"

"Polio. Both legs don't work."

"Sorry to be so nosy. I have a little brother who's got sickle cell anemia, and he's had several strokes during sickle cell crises. He's also in a wheelchair. So, I understand about that. Anything I can do, just say so."

"Thanks Adam. I've gotten adept at a lot of things. But new things always pop up. I hope I don't have to take you up on your offer, but it's nice to know you're available."

"Gotta run. New admission to work up. See ya later."

Ben heard a beep-beep-beep on his pager. He spun his chair around and spotted a phone. He picked up the phone to get his message.

"Dr. Levinson, Dr. Howard said to take the rest of the day off. Things are quiet, and he knows you were up most of the night. And he said Danny is doing very well."

Now that's nice. Cathy was wrong about the faculty being sadistic. They're quite considerate. Boy, these new pagers work well. I wonder if Boston Pediatric has them. I hear they started at Jewish Hospital in New York a couple of years ago. Nice that County is up to speed on this.

Ben went home to recover from his long stint on call. He knew it was only a partial reprieve from the rigors of internship. Sophie was delighted to see him.

"So great to have you home, if only for the night. How are you?" she said.

"Tired but happy. I'm liking my internship. Glad I went to County."

"Guess who I heard from today?" Sophie asked.

"Have no idea. Give me a hint."

"Sandra."

"Really? What did she want? I thought I'd never hear from her again."

"She didn't say. She gave me a telephone number you can call."

Ben waited until after dinner to call Sandra. He wanted to enjoy dinner with Sophie and Jacob.

"How's it going?" Jacob asked Ben once they were all seated in their traditional spots around the dining room table.

"Terrifically well, Dad. I'm learning so much. Tired all the time, but I'm not alone in that. Won't bore you with gory details, but I'm seeing cases like you wouldn't believe. The place is a museum of children's diseases."

"You see many gunshot cases or stabbings?" Sophie asked, twisting her napkin in her hands.

"None. Course, I'm in the pediatric rotation, and luckily for the kids, not many suffer gunshot wounds. Some do, usually stray bullets from some stupid gang war."

"How are things downtown?" Ben asked, turning to face Jacob.

"Well. One of the things about the jewelry business is that people always manage to find money to buy diamonds, rubies, sapphires, and emeralds even when their money runs short for other things. Don't understand it, but I'll take it."

"Mom, what're you doing these days?"

"Raising money for WGBH, Jewish Philanthropies and our local Service Center. Keeps me very busy, and I visit with a lot of my friends who do it too. I love feeling useful."

No one mentioned Cathy or Sandra. But Ben finished his dinner after a long conversation with his parents and repaired to his room to call Sandra. He was curious as to why she'd called.

"Hello?"

"Hi Sandra. Ben. Mom said you'd called."

"Yes, I did. Haven't heard from you for such a long time and wondered how you were. And why you haven't called me."

"I didn't know I was expected to call you. The last time you were here you said you'd come by when you could stay longer. You didn't, so I assumed you were no longer interested," Ben said, not trying to disguise his feelings of rejection. His mind flashed back to when they had broken up -- her idea -- long before his polio. "I'm aware that my disability could stand in the way of our relationship."

"I think I'd better come to see you rather than talk about this on the phone. I could come over now. Should I do that?"

"Yeah, come on over. I'm at home now and may not be here again for days or weeks depending on my schedule."

Ben wasn't anxious to see her but felt he should face this situation now rather than have it hovering over him, distracting him from more pressing claims on his time. Sandra had always been difficult. He thought she was a spoiled brat -- a princess wannabe -- and he felt lucky to be free from her. He went to the kitchen to tell Sophie she was coming and to ask her to bring her to his room.

When Sandra arrived, Sophie greeted her with a non-committal handshake and led her to Ben's room. After some social niceties, Sophie left them alone. She wasn't sure what this meeting was about but could see it was serious. Sandra gave Ben a friendly kiss on his cheek and sat down.

"I'm glad to see you!" she said, pulling her legs under her as she arranged herself on the loveseat. "Until I called, I hadn't realized how long it's been."

"It's nice to see you as well. You're looking good. Life treating you well?"

"Oh, very well indeed. I'll tell you all about it in a minute. But first, let me address what you said about your disability standing in the way of our relationship. You are someone I care about."

"Well, caring about another person is fine, but, really, you can't claim my paralysis doesn't alter things. And since I hadn't heard from you for so damned long, I naturally assumed it had changed things. You apparently expected me to call you, for God's sake, but somehow, strange to say, I didn't know that responsibility was mine alone. It's a two-way street, you know." Ben was still smarting from her inattention and justifiably, in his mind attributed it to his paralysis. He'd given up on her and forced her out of his mind after the long silence since her last visit.

Sandra was non-plussed about Ben's anger as her eyebrows rose and her pupils dilated.

"I can only say I was so preoccupied with my career that time went by without my noticing."

Ben looked at her incredulously. "You must have been very preoccupied with your work," he said sarcastically. "It's been several months since I've heard a word from you."

"I was definitely absorbed, believe me," she said, oblivious to his annoyance. She paused and changed tone. "I want to tell you my good news. I've been offered a faculty position at the Conservatory. Isn't that great? I'm making so much progress with my piano and conducting work, you just wouldn't believe it. I'm so excited. I've made a couple of recordings and have been asked to play at some local libraries."

Ben sat and marveled as she prattled on about her brilliant career.

"And another thing," she went on. "The dean at the Conservatory is seeking an endowment for me to be division chair. He really likes me!" She kept on jabbering, not noticing Ben's increasing anger just having her in his room.

Finally, after listening to her self-regarding monologue, he saw again that he'd been in a relationship with someone in love with only herself.

He also awoke to the pleasant fact that he would no longer be compelled to listen to her piano performances and give her over-the-top praise for her playing.

"Sandra, you haven't changed a bit. You're still so self-absorbed you haven't been interested enough in me to inquire about what I've been doing. You say you care about me. You clearly care only about yourself!" he said in a loud voice.

"There you go again, criticizing me, just like you used to do! You always find fault with me! I remember now why I wanted to break up with you!"

"Listen to me," Ben said in a calmer voice. "I'm not who I was. I can't walk. I'm wheelchair bound. I'm unable to perform sexually," he lied.

"I don't think we should continue this relationship. We're very different now than when we first began seeing each other, what was it, four years ago? First off, I'm not a musician and I don't fit into your crowd." He continued in a staccato cadence: "You have your career. I'd be an impediment to your pursuit of recognition as a top pianist or conductor. I couldn't be with you when you're on tour or attend your performances because of my obligation to patients.

"It should come as no surprise to you, but I have my own career and life. I'm committed to medicine, and I doubt you'll ever understand putting my dedication to providing service above all else.

"Right now, for example, I'm on every other night at the hospital during my internship and then there's two more years of training. That's not a life you would relish. You used to complain I was ignoring you because of my profession. It'll only get worse."

Sandra sat there simmering, absorbing all this without blinking. Ben couldn't read her reaction. Finally, she spoke.

"I'm stunned and hurt. I thought we could patch things up and go on."

"Are you kidding? No, Sandra. I'm not even sorry. It won't work."

She picked up her purse, stood up, whirled around, and left. Just like that. She didn't say goodbye, go to hell, or anything. Just left. Ben took in a deep breath, exhaled, and then inexplicably, began weeping, washing away his long-repressed anger at Sandra for both her past rejection and her more recent self-deception of her relationship with him.

Sophie knocked on the door. "Come in."

"Sandra just breezed by me and left," Sophie said, perplexed. "Didn't say a word. Want to tell me what happened?"

"We broke up. Or, I should say, I told her it was over."

"Oh."

"It just wouldn't work. For all kinds of reasons. I don't want to discuss it right now. It's a loss, but one that had to happen."

"Okay, but if any time you want to talk about it…"

"Thanks, Mom. I'm tired now. See you in the morning if you're up. I'll be leaving around six. Thanks for dinner," he said looking up into her concerned face. Seeing her worry he said, "Everything's okay. I love you. Say goodnight to Dad for me."

Chapter 23

Such Cases, August 1953

His exhaustion from work wasn't sufficient to ensure a good night's sleep. The encounter with Sandra kept his brain buzzing well past midnight. *Was ending their relationship with such finality the right thing to do?* Thinking back on his behavior, his words and tone may have been too harsh. This ambivalence kept him moving about most of the night. When dawn came, he clumsily got ready to return to the hospital for another taxing day that would extend through the night. At least working would force him to lay aside his feelings.

On the way to the hospital Ben tuned into the news. He'd remembered that Eisenhower said during his presidential campaign that he would "go to Korea." In late July an armistice was signed between North and South Korea slicing the country in two at its midsection. Now continued unrest kept the two Koreas off balance and there was constant worry that renewed conflict would ensue

In sports news, his beloved Red Sox, the only baseball team left in Boston since the Braves left Boston for Milwaukee in late 1952, lost to the Detroit Tigers on Sunday by one run. Still, they remained in fourth place in the American League. The Yankees were again on course to win the American League pennant with their all-star cast beginning with Mickey Mantle, Yogi Berra, Billy Martin and their manager, the inimitable Casey Stengel.

"Damned Yankees! We can't catch up to them," Ben said to the windshield. "We've lost the Braves, the Red Sox lost Dom DiMaggio to retirement. The only bright spot is our pitcher, Mel Parnell, who can pitch like no one else. Well, they're still fun to watch and they're above .500, so who knows what can happen in a long season? Just wish I had time to go to a game at Fenway."

Then he thought with regret, *could I navigate getting into the stands, finding a seat on those steep inclines? Where would I park my wheelchair and still have a good view of the game? And what if I had to go to the men's room? I can't stand up at a urinal anymore. Most people would never understand problems like this. I may never again get to see a baseball game at Fenway Park.*

He nosed his bulky Suburban into his designated narrow, unpaved, and rutted parking space at the hospital next to the Flannigan pavilion. The tight space made it difficult to lift his legs out of the car, get leg braces around his knees, then use his unwieldy crutches to unload the wheelchair. Anger rose as he contemplated his situation, but before he descended into one of his black moods, he reminded himself that he had a reserved parking place. For most people, parking around Suffolk County Hospital was a nightmare since it was well-nigh impossible to find a space, especially in snowy weather. Parking in the neighborhood overnight, an obvious necessity for him, also carried the risk of losing your tires or even your car to thieves. Some of the worries Jacob and Sophie had about County Hospital were based in reality.

On rounds, he focused intently on the patient updates. He'd been off duty for 48 hours, an eternity in the rapid changes of patients' conditions. The ER was quiet this Monday morning, but he knew that could change instantly. Danny, the near-drowning victim he'd admitted, had improved quickly and had already been discharged.

After rounds, he wound his stethoscope around his shoulders, checked his Harriett Lane manual, and went to the staff breakroom. Fellow interns Neil and Richard were there, looking haggard and worn after a full day and night at work.

"How was the weekend?" Ben asked.

"Last night was not bad, but Saturday was a bear. We had burns, falls, and it seemed a like a hundred diarrhea cases. Salmonella is making the rounds through Roxbury for sure," Neil said. "One of the burn cases bothers me. Take a look at this kid when you go on the ward. A four-month-old with immersion burns on his butt, uniform in depth and distribution with clear demarcation lines on the edges. Mom's accusing her live-in boyfriend of intentionally holding him down in a tub of extremely hot water as punishment for dirtying his diaper repeatedly. No splash marks around the burns, which would be expected if the child had not been held down. The poor baby probably was stooling so much because of salmonella diarrhea going around. I'd like to nail the SOB with my hockey stick." He paused, shaking his head. "We called the Department of Social Services and someone from there will interview the boyfriend and decide whether to get the police involved."

Richard now spoke up. "Then there's this other case of a four-month-old boy who allegedly fell off a couch, but his injuries are much more severe than just falling that short distance from a couch to the floor. Looks to me like the baby got slammed into a hard surface causing an occipital fracture three inches long in the back of his head. You ever heard of shaken baby syndrome? One of the attendings said he's been reading about this newly described entity. It causes blood in the subdural space and widespread retinal hemorrhages in both eyes. The neurosurgeons are getting portable x-rays of other parts of his body to rule out other fractures and then will decide if they need to operate to reduce the brain swelling and evacuate the blood. DSS is involved in this one too."

"Who brought him in?" Ben asked.

"Mom did. She's the one who said he fell off the couch."

"Did the social worker find anything else from the mom?"

"She was evasive, the social worker said. You don't know who's to blame. When DSS gets further along, maybe we'll know more. I sure hope so. That kid shouldn't go back to that home, in my opinion."

"Wow," Ben said. "Sorry I missed seeing those cases. But I don't know if I'd keep my head dealing with people who did that. How can they do that?"

"Beats me. It was all I could do to keep from telling the mother I thought she was a damned liar, that those injuries couldn't possibly happen from falling off a couch. Our attending scoffed too when he heard the story, sarcastically labelling it the "killer couch." But you never know what mom's living with either. Maybe she's getting beaten up too. The attending said he'd seen other cases like this. What I don't understand is why I never heard anything about child abuse in medical school. It never came up in any of my lectures. I wonder how frequent it is."

"Somebody must have stats on that. DSS maybe. I'm gonna look into it," Ben said.

As the weeks went by, Ben could hardly believe the diversity of cases he saw. After his time in the emergency room, he rotated to the inpatient service where he was nearly overwhelmed with anemias whose origins were diverse, all the way from simple iron deficiency through thalassemia, sickle cell, aplastic anemia, and early leukemia. There were also infectious diseases -- meningitis, sepsis, pneumonia, croup, epiglottitis, and the disease Ben was all too familiar with, polio. These cases, many left-over from the summer were varied, with paralyses of muscles ranging from the face, upper arms, and legs. Some needed assisted ventilation in the iron lung to survive.

He saw kidney diseases from a variety of causes, heart diseases, both congenital and resulting from diseases. He was seeing so many pediatric conditions that he nearly wore out the 900 pages of Nelson's pediatrics textbook. He wondered if he'd ever be able to know enough to be confident in his diagnosis and treatment decisions.

Time was passing so fast it was like being on a toboggan ride down a steep hill. Fall came to Boston, with kids grudgingly returning to school, happily trading germs with each other. The pediatric emergency room was abuzz with coughs, runny noses, rashes, sore throats, and fevers. There were traumatic injuries of all kinds, belly aches, and a plethora of ear infections. Mixed in with these mostly acute, non-life-threatening conditions, were sneaky diagnostic problems that turned out to be serious diseases. These were admitted to the inpatient service for consultation with subspecialists requiring the interns to do a dizzying number of blood tests, X-rays, and more complex diagnostic testing.

More than once, Ben met parents who gave him suspicious attention when they were confronted by a doctor in a wheelchair. But once he worked with them, they became convinced of his competence, his empathy, and his total involvement in caring for their child. It was hard for Ben, though, and it took time for him to get over his resentment of their skepticism. He tried telling himself that their reaction was one that he himself might have had before this had happened to him.

~~~

"Where you goin' for the holidays?" Adam Fisher asked Ben at Billy's sandwich shop where they often went for lunch, a couple of streets away from the hospital. Nobody could stand the wretched food in the hospital cafeteria, which not only served putrid food, but the place smelled rancid and looked dirty.

"Need to check with family and my girlfriend," Ben said. "Being Jewish I always work the Christmas holidays in place of my Christian colleagues. Then I usually get time off for Thanksgiving."

"Girlfriend? Well, now, you've never told me about her," Adam said with a wide smile.

"I don't tell you everything," Ben laughed. "It's early in our relationship, but I think it's the real thing."
~~~

"Well, congratulations! And good luck," he said, looking at Ben inquisitively.

"I know what you're thinking, you bad son of a minister," Ben chuckled. "The answer is 'yes' but you better not say anything to anyone, or I'll have to kill you."

"Good for you. I'm happy for you. But remember what the attendings say: When you're an intern, you may as well put your balls on ice."

"I bet they didn't do that when they were interns. 'Do as I say, not as I did.' So, where are you going on vacation?"

"Probably home. Dad can't get away and I wanna see him and Mom, so Cambridge Maryland is probably where I'll be."

"Why can't he get away?"

"Upcoming holidays are always a busy time for him. Especially for the AME."

"Fill me in. What's AME?"

"African Methodist Episcopalian. Sort of a hybrid Protestant sect. Prevalent in Maryland. The Methodist part comes from the fact that Methodists were abolitionists. And Cambridge was part of the Underground Railway during those bad years. Harriet Tubman was active there for a time, part of the Underground Railroad."

"Interesting. Ever consider going into the ministry?"

"I considered it, but I figured I could help people more by ministering to their bodies in the here and now. Dad, on the other hand, is deeply committed to saving souls in his community. It takes a toll on him."

"How so?"

"He gets discouraged often when his people get hurt by racists. Maryland's really a Southern state." He considered what he'd just said. "That's not to say that racism is confined to the South. But it's rampant in Maryland. Watching my dad agonize over some of his congregant's problems helped me decide to be a doctor. Seems to me it's a more concrete way of helping people. And a doctor can try to heal both physical and emotional ailments. So, we'll see."

Adam looked at his watch. "I got a patient coming in five minutes. Mind if I go on ahead?"

"No, go ahead. See you back there."

"Sure you don't need any help?"

"No, I'll be fine. I'm just kinda slow on the uneven sidewalks. Thanks anyway."

Adam hurried away. Ben paid Billy for lunch and began wheeling himself on a street parallel to Massachusetts Avenue. He looked at the wasteland of vacant lots that were cleared several years ago for a building project that never came to pass, noticing broken bottles, cans, fragments of bricks, vinyl siding, discarded tires, newspapers and other trash of all descriptions, symbols of neglect of inner cities occurring in communities everywhere in the country.

As he contemplated this, he became aware of a couple of early teens -- colored boys -- approaching him. He tried to be nonchalant, but as they came closer, he knew they were up to no good. His heart rate picked up and despite the cool weather, he broke out in a cold sweat.

"Empty your pockets, white cracker," one of them said, trying to be menacing. "Put all you stuff in this bag," holding a paper bag in front of his chair. Ben was terrified, but he tried to put on a brave front.

"And what if I don't?"

One of the pair pulled out a kitchen knife and said, "See this?"

"Yeah, I see it." Ben stared at the gleaming metal blade, wondering how he was going to survive, even if he gave up his wallet to these hoodlums. He reached back to get his wallet to comply with the order to toss it into the bag. The boy moved closer with the knife.

"Don't try anything, white boy, or you'll be sorry."

"You asked for my wallet and I'm just getting it out."

"Better not be anything else you gettin' out," the one with the knife said. "Else you be dead!"

Out of the corner of his eye Ben was surprised to see Adam coming up on them from behind. What's he doing here?

"Hey! Hey! Hey!! Back off, you two, and fast, or you'll have to deal with me!" Adam shouted with authority in his deep bass voice.

The boys' eyes widened, and they stepped back, seeing this six-foot two man with upper arms as big as their thighs. They knew he meant business.

"Get your sorry asses away from him. This man is a doctor at the hospital and my good friend," he lectured the stunned and frightened teens, "and you two better clear out before I clear y'all out for good. Didn't your mama ever teach you anything? You get on outta here, now, go!!"

The boys, confronted with the reality of their situation, ran off, looking back furtively over their shoulders at this guy who materialized out of nowhere.

Ben looked at Adam. "Wow! My bodyguard. Thanks! What made you come back?"

"My patient didn't show, so I thought I'd come and walk you back. Good thing I did, huh?"

"Boy, you bet. You sure scared those two off. You even scared me a little," he laughed.

"They're just dumb kids, trying out to be men, but the wrong kind," Adam said. "Pitiful. They probably watch a lot of TV, see all these action heroes pushing people around. And some macho guys in their neighborhood. They're led on by all that trash on TV to believe that's what men are 'sposed to be. They think bullying people will prove their manhood. Too bad. They're probably good kids, just misguided and impressionable. I'll give you 100 to 1 odds they have no fathers around. They have no proper role models.

"I doubt they'd have followed through with the knife because they're so young and scared themselves, but I wasn't gonna take the chance."

"Well, thanks, Adam. But when you come to my house, don't mention this to my folks. This kind of thing was their worst fear when I signed on here at County. I don't want to raise their anxiety level any higher."

"I promise. Let's get back to the hospital. I expect you have patients too. My next patient will probably be there. Unless they don't show either. A lot of my patients have transportation problems and don't have phones to cancel their appointments. Common problem with inner city folks. Then they get blamed for being irresponsible parents. They can't win."

Ben thought about what just happened.

"I'm learning new things every day I work in this neighborhood," he said. "Things that have nothing to do with medicine, but with poverty, racial tensions, crime, poor parenting, and a multitude of other societal issues. But I'm also learning about resiliency. Most people just trying to live their lives, raise their families, get their kids the education they need. And you're helping me learn, Adam. I appreciate that more than you can know."

Chapter 24

Thanksgiving with the Levinsons

"What time will Cathy be coming?" Sophie asked Ben, as she raced around the dining room, fussing over details of napkins, plates, and silverware.

"Around 10. She wanted to come in time to give you a hand."

"I wonder how we'll get along," she said as she reset the table a third time, arranging cut flowers in different places each time. "After the Sandra saga, I don't know how to act with your girlfriends."

"Mom, settle down. You'll be fine. You and she will hit it off from the first moment. She's so easy to know. You'll see."

Jacob walked in and looked around.

"Anything I can do?" he said, knowing the answer was "no" since Sophie preferred getting everything ready for dinners by herself.

"You can light some logs in the fireplace," she said turning, dropping a teacup, shattering it on the floor.

"Oh drats!" she cried, "Could you get the broom and dustpan for me?"

"Sophie, why don't you take a break? It's early and festivities won't start for another few hours," Jacob said, as he cleaned up the breakage and took Sophie in his arms, comforting her.

Ben could see he was of no use and moved into his room, leaving the door open. He put on music that filled not only his room but flowed into the dining room.

By the time Cathy arrived, Sophie's nervousness had subsided, and she was her usual gracious self. After introductions, they all gathered in the library to get more acquainted.

"So, Cathy," Jacob said warmly, "fill Sophie and me in about yourself."

"Um, well, I'm a nurse, but I guess you already know that," she smiled. She told them about growing up in Southie and the other things she had told Ben.

"Ben may have told us but remind me how you two first met," Sophie said.

"Well, I first noticed Ben when he was a medical student on pediatrics, and I was a nurse on the ward. But he didn't know I was staring at him," she said with a faint blush. "Later, I worked on the floor when he was sick. An awkward moment for both of us. I was flustered because I hadn't been able to get him out of my mind since I first saw him, don't know why, exactly. He seemed a little embarrassed too. I could tell because he got a little red when I lowered my mask to reveal my face -- at his request, I must add -- and we both were sort of self-conscious. I didn't see him again for a long time. Then, all of a sudden, when I was getting off an elevator at Pediatric Hospital, I saw him on his way to his intern interview."

"What has he told you about his difficult parents?" Jacob asked smiling.

"That you're just awful people," she laughed. "Seriously, and I'm not making this up, everything he's told me made me want to meet you. Thanks for inviting me."

"We're so glad you could come," Sophie said. "You know, Thanksgiving is my favorite holiday. It has nothing to do with religions, no gifts are expected, and except for preparing dinner, it's easy to host."

"Your home is so lovely. And dinner smells so good!" Cathy said. "I live over a restaurant, and I'm treated to great food smells all the time. Has Ben told you about my apartment?"

"Only that it's as you said, over an Ethiopian restaurant in Jamaica Plain. How long have you been there?" Sophie asked.

"A couple of years. As it turns out, it's a great place to live during my fellowship at Channing. I can walk there, except when it's bad weather."

"What are you studying at Channing?" Jacob asked.

"Community health. The mechanics of bringing health care to underserved communities. Very interesting, and I think, very important."

"How long is your fellowship?" Sophie inquired.

"Probably two years. But it depends on whether I want to go on to get a PhD or only a master's degree."

"I hope she goes on for her PhD since I won't finish my residency for three years," Ben said.

Sophie sensed this segment of conversation was over, and said, "Have you seen Ben's room? We're very proud of what we did to make it work for him."

"Let's wait until after dinner. I'm starved!" Ben said.

"Okay, dinner is served!" They all moved into the dining room and enjoyed a typical American Thanksgiving, complete with Jacob talking about the mythology about the first Thanksgiving. After dinner they toured the rest of the house and ended up in Ben's room.

"Boy, this is so well done," she enthused. "You're so lucky to have this place, Ben."

"I'm very grateful to these two. My awful parents," he teased. They went back to the library for after-dinner tea, then relaxed and watched Thanksgiving Day football games.

They enjoyed each other's company, but all were exquisitely aware of sensitive issues in this evolving relationship: first, what Ben's paralysis would auger for their future and second, their disparate religious and family backgrounds. But none wanted to touch those delicate subjects, not even to nibble around the edges. These were four adults who were proving to be masters of avoidance of pressing issues in their lives. It was like a crowd of people in Grand Central Station ignoring a naked man walking through the terminal. The family's confrontation with reality would come at another time, another place.

Chapter 25

The Fall

For those who desired a white Christmas, the snowfall was a welcome event. For many men, it was more a curse than a blessing. Shoveling snow for them gave rise to strained backs, sore arms, falls, and, in worst case scenarios, heart attacks.

For Ben, it was a near disaster when he slipped and fell on black ice under the flaky snow in his parking space beside the Flannigan pavilion. He landed hard on his left outstretched arm. First, he felt pain in his shoulder and then, his paralysis made it impossible to move and gain an upright position.

When Dr. Sullivan, who had a parking space next to Ben's, discovered him on the ground, the mid-twenties temperature had rendered him hypothermic, in great pain and confused. Sullivan immediately got him into the emergency department where they wrapped him in warm blankets, took his vital signs, gave him medicine for pain and obtained X-rays of his upper body, focusing on his left shoulder and left arm.

By the time he got to the radiology suite, he'd regained some awareness of his surroundings. He knew Becca, the X-ray technician.

"I'm so mad at myself. I should slow down and be more careful," he complained.

"Come on, don't blame yourself," Becca said. "You're the third fall case I've seen here this morning. People fall when there's snow. See it all the time."

"I was supposed to be on duty upstairs an hour ago. Can someone call and let them know I'm here?"

"We already did. They said to tell you not to worry, someone is covering for you."

"How can I work the holidays if I'm in a cast or something?"

"Cross that bridge later."

"Oh, by the way, did someone bring my wheelchair in?"

"Yeah, it's in the ER. Dr. Sullivan brought it in. As far as working is concerned, you won't be able to until after they get this shoulder attended to."

"What do you see on the films?"

"Not developed yet. Besides, I can't tell you anything. I'm only a tech."

"I bet you can read X-rays as well as the radiologists, with all your experience."

"I can see the obvious things, but not borderline findings. The radiologists are terrific here. Every time I get to thinking I can read films they find something I didn't even see."

Back in the Emergency Room, Dr. Matt told Ben, "Well, you dislocated your shoulder, but luckily no fractures, and the rotator cuff, as best as we can tell, is intact."

"Good. Means I can go back to work? I hate letting the team down."

"Nope. You need time for your shoulder to calm down. Maybe a week. Besides, you can't propel yourself around in your wheelchair with a bum shoulder. Also, I heard you drive an assisted car, right? Your left shoulder won't allow you to do that."

"Yeah, all true. You're right, of course. How'd you know about the car?"

"Dr. Sullivan told us he'd looked for your wheelchair and noticed the special levers you have on the driver's side. As far as your letting the team down, look at it this way," Matt said. "During the course of a year almost all interns are out of commission a while, for some reason. This is your time. Once you rehab that shoulder, you'll be ready to roll."

Ben used the ER phone to call home.

"Mom? Me. Just listen without interrupting me," he said, trying to keep Sophie from panicking. "First thing, I'm perfectly okay, but I fell this morning and dislocated my shoulder."

"Oh, no, Benji," she gasped. "You say you're okay, but are you really?"

"Yeah, I'm fine, in the ER at the hospital. What? Suffolk County Hospital, of course. No, no, I'm fine here. Here's the thing. I obviously can't drive so I need you to come get me. Okay?"

"Be right there. Where shall I come? Where will I find you?"

"Drive into the ambulance entrance. I'll be at the door of the adult ER in my chair. The aides will help get me into your car. You and Dad will need to come back later to get the Suburban. I'll show you where it's parked."

The pickup went smoothly. Ben showed Sophie where his car was, and when they got home two high school neighbor boys, out of school for the holidays, helped him into the house. Once the flurry of activity getting him in the house and situated in the kitchen was past, Sophie gave him lunch and called Jacob. Ben called Cathy and left a message at the public health school for her to call him at home.

Over a late lunch Ben told Sophie how he'd slipped on the ice and fallen, the ensuing adventure on the ground and what happened in the ER.

"Could have happened to anybody," he said, trying to convince her it was no big deal.

"Yes, but when things like that happen to you, it's not the same to me. So, you're my prisoner until I tell you you're free," she said with a smile, "I'm going to be a real Jewish mother until you're completely well."

Ben knew he had little choice when his mother made this kind of declaration. He sighed and finished his sandwich.

"I called Cathy, but I haven't heard back. Hope she can come over this evening. Is that okay?"

"Of course. She could come for dinner if she's free. You have anything you'd like for dinner? I'm going to the store soon as I clean up after lunch."

"Whatever you'd like to make. I'm glad to be home."

~~~

Cathy arrived at the Levinson's home around six by cab. Jacob, who had come home right after Sophie told him about Ben's accident, was filled in on all the details when Sophie drove him back to the hospital parking lot to get the Suburban. When Jacob got back and walked into the kitchen, he saw everyone hugging one another. "Should I get in line?"

Cathy laughed and gave him a big hug as well.

"Well, Ben, you sure know how to get attention!" Jacob said. "How're you feeling by now?"

"I'm ready to go back to work, but she," pointing to Sophie, "won't let me do anything. Tell her to back off!"

"You're asking the wrong guy," Jacob laughed. "She never listens to me."

"Let's eat, I'm famished," Ben said.

After dinner, they lingered and talked a while, but soon Sophie shooed Ben and Cathy into Ben's room, knowing they yearned to be together. Sophie and Jacob
~~~

left them alone for a couple of hours, then knocked on his door.

"Come in," Cathy called out.

"We're going up to bed. Anything you need?" Sophie said.

"No thanks. Cathy needs to get going soon anyway," Ben said.

"Did they give you anything for pain?" Sophie asked.

"Yeah, already took it. I feel okay now," he said, winking at Cathy.

"Goodnight, both of you. What did they tell you about a follow-up visit?"

"Tomorrow, in the orthopedic clinic at two. Can you take me?"

"Sure. See you in the morning."

"You want to stay the night?" Ben asked Cathy after Sophie left.

"Well, I'd like to, but I don't think your folks are quite ready for that. I can just see the expression on your mother's face if she sees me here in the morning," Cathy said with a big grin. "I've already called a cab."

"Can you come again tomorrow night?"

"Sure."

"I can suggest they go out to a movie, and you can have your way with me," Ben said, a smile spreading across his face.

"You think we could get away with that?" she said, interested in the idea.

"Yup. We could even do it now if you're game."

"Uh, no, don't think we should. Sorry to be a prude. I love you though." She gave him a prolonged deep kiss, and Ben tried to pull her closer but grimaced in pain.

"Damn, you made me forget all about my shoulder. Worth it, though."

"See you tomorrow. Hope you can sleep."

She left but the sweet smell of her hair lingered in the air. Ben smiled at his good fortune.

~~~

Jacob watched Sophie as she prepared herself for bedtime. Her routine had been unvaried for years, consisting of applying cold cream to her face, leaving it on while she brushed her teeth, slipping into her nightgown, taking off the cold cream with tissues, then nestling into bed with a yawn. She usually was asleep within minutes, but tonight she lay awake.

"What's on your mind?" Jacob asked.

"Well, what do you think would be on my mind after the last couple of days?" she said irritably.

"Do you mean Ben's accident or his girlfriend?"

"You must be mind reader," Sophie said, turning to face Jacob who had gotten into bed next to her.

"Well, which is topmost in your mind?"

"I guess the latter. His shoulder will heal. I don't know what to think about his relationship with Cathy."
~~~

"I'm also concerned."

"Is it that she's not Jewish?"

"Of course, that's one concern, but I'm also perplexed about her interest in Ben. It's not natural for a young, attractive girl like Cathy to want a relationship with, uh, well, I don't know how else to put it, a crippled man."

"Yes. That's it. I'm torn, because I think he really, I don't know, can I say loves her, or at least likes her a lot. She seems to return his affection, but why? I love Ben, he's my son. I hate myself for thinking he's not lovable by a woman, but the reality is that he's not, you know, a young man who can go hiking, skiing, play tennis, and so forth."

They lay silent for a few moments, these thoughts suspended in the darkness of the room.

"The shicksa thing is another worry for me," Sophie finally said, raising this sensitive issue. "I know the Sandra affair put a damper on Ben's attitude toward women in general and Jewish women in particular. He talked to me about that when he broke off with Sandra. But getting involved with an Irish Catholic girl from Southie is the ultimate departure from what I'd hoped would happen. I don't know. I try not to be judgmental but, with all that's happened to our people, it's hard not to have strong opinions about trusting outsiders."

"I think of our decision to leave Germany, all those years ago, because of antisemitism and the rise of Nazism," Jacob said. "I wonder what Abraham would say. I don't really know, I can only guess. But this bothers me. And I don't know how to bring up my concern with Ben. Do you?"

"No. We've raised him in the Jewish tradition, although we're not what you'd call real observant Jews. But we're living in 1950's America. It's confusing, and frustrating, to know what's right. You know we'll have to confront this sometime. This can't go unaddressed. We also don't know a thing about Cathy's family's attitude about her going with a Jew, but my guess is they don't like the idea."

"Worry never helps solve problems," Jacob said. "Let's try to get some sleep. Problems always seem worse at night." He leaned over and gave Sophie a goodnight kiss. But neither slept well that night.

Chapter 26

Lead Poisoning

The orthopedic clinic was packed the next day. Ben was not alone in sustaining an injury because of the snow. He looked around at his fellow patients and they were of all ages, all colors, all nationalities, and the cacophony of diverse languages was deafening. He wished he'd paid more attention in his high school language classes because his patients might speak in any of the various dialects of Spanish, French or Portuguese, in addition to ghetto talk. He learned some by osmosis but was glad hospital interpreters were available to help him grasp their descriptions of what ailed them, then translate his advice.

In addition to the languages redolent of the tower of Babel, multiple odors hung in the air. Simple sweat was the most identifiable, but also in the mix were odors of food—fish, garlic, onions, meats -- being consumed by patients in the waiting room. The smell of strong perfumes competing with ammoniacal odor of urine, and the sulphury smell of stool emanated from some. This miasma was more pronounced here in this clinic serving adults than Ben encountered in pediatric clinics, where the predominant odors were from unchanged cloth diapers.

"Ben Levinson!" cried the nurse. He moved his wheelchair through the crowded room following the nurse into the exam room. She took his vital signs quickly and left.

Hmm. Pretty cold nurse. No personality. But what did I expect? Red carpets because I'm a white doctor? I'm sure she doesn't know I'm a doctor. How would she know? Maybe she's having a bad day. Maybe all days are bad for her. Really getting to know people around here is not as easy as in my Brookline neighborhood or as it was with my fellow medical students. I expect some are fighting personal battles. So, I should be kind. Give them the benefit of the doubt.

The door opened and a tall athletic man about Ben's age came in.

"Hi, I'm Dr. Charley Duncan. Understand you're a pediatric intern here. I'm a resident. Glad to meet you," offering his hand.

Ben shook his hand, meeting his gaze. "Ben Levinson. Good to meet you, although I'd rather have met you over lunch," he smiled.

"How's the shoulder feeling today?"

"Not bad."

"Let me see you raise your arm over your head."

Ben grimaced as he did this. "Hurts but doesn't kill me."

"Taking any meds?"

"A little aspirin. Don't think I need anything stronger."

"Okay. Well, you're lucky. I think with some exercises we should be able to get you back in commission soon."

He showed Ben some exercises and sent him on his way. He met Sophie in the waiting room, and they left for the car.

"Whew, glad to be out of that smelly place," Sophie said.

"Still wish you'd taken your training at Pediatric Hospital."

"I knew you'd say that, but this is where I decided to come," Ben said with an edge. "It may take some getting used to it for you and Dad, but I'm happy I'm here. I'm learning more than medicine."

Sophie remained silent until they were a few blocks up Massachusetts Avenue.

"What did they say about your shoulder?"

He told her about the exercises Dr. Duncan prescribed as they drove home.

"When can you get back to being an intern?"

"He said about a week, depending on how I feel. I think I'll be ready to go back next Monday."

Their conversation was perfunctory, as Ben could feel Sophie's tensions about his internship at Suffolk County Hospital adding to the unspoken disquietude that he knew both Jacob and Sophie had about his evolving romance with Cathy. Sooner or later, he'd have to discuss this with them, and a similar discussion would have to take place with Cathy and her parents. To say nothing of the necessary discussion between the two sets of parents.

When they got home, he was able to get out on his own with his braces and into the wheelchair. As soon as he got in his room, he called the pediatric intern's office to tell them he would be back on Monday. He then set about doing the exercises Dr. Duncan had given him.

On rounds on Monday, Neil and Richard filled him in on all the patients.

"Meet Nell, our newest guest," Richard said as he smiled at the four-year-old colored girl in traction for a femoral fracture. "This is Dr. Ben. He fell down just like you, but he didn't break anything."

"Why's he in that wheelchair then?" Nell said in typical childlike honesty.

"That's from something else, Nell," Ben answered. "But my arm is fine," as he raised his arm over his head. "See?"

"When can I go home?" she said, ignoring Ben's demonstration.

"The bone doctors will be by soon. They're the bosses when it comes to your injury. We just wanted to say hello."

"Why is she on pediatrics?" Ben asked as they were out of earshot.

"There's some question about the mechanism of injury. It's a spiral fracture of the femur and they're checking her out for other injuries and getting the social worker involved in talking to her mother," Neil said. "The ortho team said that kind of fracture is due to a twisting of the upper leg with a lot of force. Mom said she fell in their kitchen and ortho doesn't see how that injury could have happened from a fall like that."

The next patient they saw was a three-month-old infant in a mist tent, with arms in soft restraints and an oxygen cannula in his nose. Neil kept on describing all the patients they had been seeing.

"Little guy here has bronchiolitis. He's better than when he came in. Had low oxygen sats on admission, a lot of retractions of his rib cage, but he's better today.

"Next in our parade of stars is this toddler, who got into a bottle of pills and by the time mother found him, he'd ingested, she thought, about ten of them. She had the presence of mind to bring the bottle in. It's an antibiotic mom is on for urinary tract infection, so it was not toxic. He's fine, going home this afternoon. He may get loose stools from the antibiotic. I think Mom knows now to keep all meds out of reach.

"This is Adeline," Neil said, moving on to the next bed. "She's two and a feisty little girl. She has this habit of eating peeling paint from the windowsills in her house. Apparently, this paint has a sweet taste according to her mom. When she told Dr. Chase, our chief resident, about her pica, the term used for eating non-food items like paint chips, he got X-rays of her abdomen and knees. The ends of the long bones of the legs showed growth arrest lines, also known now as 'lead lines.' The abdominal films showed a bunch of white radio-opaque shadows, most likely from the ingested paint chips.

"It's interesting that most of the highest-quality paint made before World War II was made with lead," Neil said. "Just so you don't think I'm inherently brilliant, I must tell you I went to the medical library. There I found out that chips measuring about one square centimeter from lead-based paint contain 1.5 mg or more of lead. We're waiting on her blood reports to see how high the blood lead level is."

"Been seeing much of this?" Ben asked.

"At least two to three cases each month."

"Are the paint chips the only source of lead kids can access?"

"No, lots of other places to get lead into the body," Neil went on, loving his teaching role. "Surface soil and dust from sanding or scraping of lead paint is one place. Automobile batteries all contain large amounts of lead, and one mode of disposal of these batteries is burning them.

"Well, the smoke from burning batteries makes lead airborne. Inhalation of this smoke is much worse than ingestion because the lead is more concentrated in the smoke. Also, gasoline we use every day in our cars has tetra-ethyl lead added to it, so exhaust fumes contain small amounts of lead.

"When I looked into this, I found a lot of potential lead exposure every day, especially in cities like ours. For instance, home water pipes often have lead in them. Certain glazes on pottery have lead and can leach out with acidic beverages. Even some jewelry and painted toys may have lead."

"I had no idea that lead was so ubiquitous," Ben said. "Do these kids have symptoms?"

"The majority have no symptoms until the lead levels get high. Some with high blood lead levels come in with seizures, some with abdominal pain, some have vomiting, constipation, listlessness. Some are hyperirritable. But, as I said, waiting for symptoms shouldn't be done if there's known exposure. Getting blood levels is the sine-quo-non of diagnosing lead poisoning."

"What's the usual lead level in kids?"

"Kids -- people generally -- should have zero lead in their blood. My guess is that Adeline's level will be somewhere between 40 and 80 micrograms per milliliter. That's a lot."

"So, what treatment will you use?"

"The first and foremost is to remove her from where she's getting this lead. That means getting her out of her home. That would seem obvious and easy to do, but it's not. Where will mom move to? Another old building with lead poisoning waiting to happen? And landlords can't be compelled to remove the lead under current laws. So, we're stuck in that respect.

"We can do chelation therapy. This means giving her a drug that binds the lead in the blood and causes the kidneys to excrete it. Takes time and isn't without side-effects. So, we're stuck there too. This is definitely a public health problem."

Ben was really taken by this problem. He wondered how frequent lead poisoning was, how many kids got it, and how doctors could effect some change in this multilayered disorder. And what were the implications on the long-term health of children?

"What can high blood lead levels do to kids?" Ben asked Neil, who seemed to know a lot about it.

"Impedes brain development. Not much is known, but what we do know is that it affects the brain's cognitive functions and kids who have had lead poisoning do poorly in school and have social problems -- they get labeled as 'retarded' and get teased about it by their peers."

Ben's interest picked up. His own disability made him sensitive to other forms of "differentness." This was beginning to gestate in his mind as a calling, as Uncle Abraham would have said.

He needed to find out more about whether this was even a subspecialty in pediatrics. Was anyone doing research in children's mental development? Physical development?

How many pediatric psychologists or psychiatrists are there? Who would know about such things? Maybe the Departmental Chairman could provide some answers to this.

Chapter 27

Meeting with Dr. Friedman

Ben fidgeted with his stethoscope while waiting outside Stephen Friedman's office, his Department Chairman, for a five o'clock appointment. Dr. Friedman was a noted pediatric endocrinologist whose special interest was thyroid disease. Ben was nervous because he wasn't clear what his questions should be, but he needed guidance about a focus in his training.

He'd only seen Dr. Friedman on stage in the top floor of the Flannigan Building during intern orientation, but he'd never met him face to face. This added to his uncertainty as to whether this appointment would yield anything helpful to his decision-making about his pathway in pediatrics. His faculty advisor, Dr. Makin, a pleasant older man but quite shy, seemed unduly intimidated by seeing Ben in his wheelchair. He had been of little help when he'd met with him.

The secretary called his name and ushered him into Friedman's modest office on the first floor of the Flannigan Building. He was a slight man whose wire-rimmed glasses had thick lenses like the bottoms of coke bottles, magnifying his liquid brown eyes. His shiny bald head reflected the glare of harsh fluorescent lights hanging from the ceiling. When he stood to welcome Ben, his handshake was firm. His tattersall shirt and plain brown tie rode under his unbuttoned tweed jacket that displayed a small paunch, the only clue to his middle age.

"Very glad to meet you, Ben. I've heard many good things about you. Sorry you had your recent fall but glad you're recovering so well." Ben was impressed that he knew about his fall.

"Thanks for your good wishes, sir."

He looked at Ben and asked, "What can I do for you?"

"Well, I'm groping for some direction. My first months here have shown me a lot about pediatric diseases, but more than that, I'm struck about how naive I've been about other influences on children's health," he explained. "For example, the lead poisoning patient I recently saw jolted me awake to a whole new area of concern -- environment -- on children's well-being," he said, taking a deep breath.

Aware he was going on in a rapid-fire style, he wondered if he was just babbling away, with no coherence. Nevertheless, he continued.

"I saw a couple of kids who may have been abused, another with an ingestion of mother's pills, and still another with burns. In medical school I learned about genetic syndromes, metabolic abnormalities, and congenital heart problems, but now I'm struck with these different kinds of major problems affecting large numbers of children, that I never considered because I'd never heard of them before. This year is wearing me out with all the dilemmas I'm seeing."

"Glad the scales are falling off your eyes," Friedman said with a smile. "Unfortunately, the perception of pediatricians by many is that we're just 'baby doctors' who see runny noses, coughs and diaper rashes. As you're finding out, there's so much more. Before your time, pediatrics split off from internal medicine because the things afflicting children are so different from adult diseases. Not only the negative environmental and family situations so many children live under, but the whole field of childhood infectious diseases.

"For example, we now have more and better vaccines to stop the suffering and deaths due to communicable diseases. We need to do a much better job of telling these stories. It's only when an epidemic hits us that people pay attention to what pediatrics has done for disease prevention." He paused, realizing he was preaching to the choir. Shifting gears abruptly, he said, "So, what do you see yourself doing in pediatrics?"

"Well, a number of things," Ben began. "I enjoy being around medical students and hope I can pass on whatever knowledge I have to them. So, I'm thinking I want to teach, maybe in medical school, but surely in the hospital. I see a need to ensure better care for the poor. Those cases of lead poisoning and child abuse and other childhood accidental ingestions shook me. I think these things need to be studied in more detail and programs need to be designed and implemented to address them."

"These are just the tip of that iceberg," Friedman said. "I think what you're describing -- the whole iceberg, so to speak -- is what is starting to be called community or social pediatrics. It's public health cum preventive medicine cum social awareness. It's meeting the diverse needs of communities, both large and small."

"The other area I'm interested in, for obvious reasons, are disabilities," Ben said. "Physical limitations, for sure, like mine, but also people with developmental and psychological handicaps. There are so many problems, beginning with adverse birth events, but continuing through a multitude of childhood illnesses, accidental and non-accidental injuries, and on and on," he trailed off.

"The immensity of needs seems overwhelming at times," Ben said. "Then there's sleep deprivation. Every other night on call is bad even for those who aren't in a wheelchair. I hope I can make it through without total exhaustion."

"Internship will end," Friedman said. "I know it doesn't seem that way while you're in the middle of it. Hang in there, you'll make it.

"As to the other things you brought up. I think you're on the right wavelength, Ben. Your enthusiasm is there, motivation is there, your passion is there, and, importantly, your brainpower is evident. Let's talk from time to time to keep you on an even keel towards these goals. I can see you as a future chief resident and later as a faculty member. I'm glad you came to see me," he said, bringing the conversation to an end.

Ben left Dr. Friedman's office wanting to shout "hallelujah" but he simply smiled broadly all the way to his car. When he got home, he told Sophie all about his conversation with enormous enthusiasm.

"That's so great, Benji. Glad you went to see him. Maybe County Hospital is the right place for you, after all," she laughed, and Ben was pleased she could finally see a good side of his chosen hospital. When Jacob got home and Ben told him how excited he was, he also was pleased that Ben was finding something he could believe in.

After dinner, Ben called Cathy.

"Hi. I miss you. When can we get together?"

"Your call. It's easier for me to find time. Your schedule doesn't really care much about us, you know?"

"I know. I can't do anything about that, as you know. Next year it will be only every third night, not every other night.

"I wanted to tell you about my meeting with Dr. Friedman, my departmental chairman." He summarized his session with Friedman, embellishing it to some degree by his passion. At the end, he waited for her reaction.

"I'm glad you talked to him. I don't know him, obviously, but it seems apparent why he's the chairman of the department. He sounds terrific. I hope to meet him some day."

"I have to make up for my absences at work because of my fall, so I can't get away until next weekend. Are you available to have me come to your place Sunday after next?"

"Sounds good," Cathy said. "I've missed you so much."

"Me too. You haven't found another guy because of your absentee lover?"

"You're so silly sometimes, Ben. Jealousy doesn't become you, especially since you have no competition." They both were quiet for a moment, then Cathy said, "What do you think about meeting my parents?"

"Scares me, but I know it's something I've got to do. You survived meeting mine, so I guess I can do likewise. When?"

"I'll check with them and let you know. We ought to meet them at their place. Do you think you want the whole family, or just the two of them?"

"Oh, boy, I'd like to take it slow and easy, just them at first. What do you think?"

"Yeah, I think that's best. I'll work on it. Call me tomorrow. I love you."

"Love you too."

He hung up and his anxiety grew as he thought about Mr. and Mrs. Kelly. *When I think of them, all the stereotypes of Southie flood into my mind. Racists. Jew-haters. Alcoholics. Blond, blue eyed people. Redheads with freckles. Shanty Irish. Lace curtain Irish. Northern Ireland hatreds. On and on. Got to wash those things out of my mind. Remember Cathy and how much she means to me.*

Chapter 28

Meg and Jack Kelly

The die was cast. They would meet with the Kelly's at their house in a month on a Sunday afternoon. Ben wanted to talk to Susan Goodall, the social worker he knew from his time in Boston Pediatric Hospital. He hoped she could talk to him or see him. Maybe she had a private practice outside of the hospital. He called Dr. Weller's office the next day between patients and was pleased that Ellie answered.

"Ben Levinson, what a pleasure to hear from you. How're you doing?"

"Doing well. Extremely well, in fact. But I need to talk to Susan Goodall, the social worker I met when I was an inpatient. Do you know how I can reach her?"

"I'll find her telephone number. I'll also tell Dr. Weller you called. And if you're ever in the neighborhood, we'd both be glad to see you!"

He was surprised when Susan answered after the first ring.

"Hello, Ben," she said. "Ellie called and told me you wanted to talk. How're you doing?"

"Very well, thanks. No problem with my health, just need some of your good advice. Is there some time we could talk? Either by phone or in person?"

"Sure. My guess is your time is tighter than mine. When can you talk?"

"If you're free now, that'd be great. Or I can call you back."

"Fire away. I don't have any patients until after lunch. You know, morning rounds with the medical team puts my other work off till afternoons."

"Well, here's the thing. I've met a wonderful woman, Cathy Kelly's her name, and I'm about to meet her parents. Cathy's part of a large Irish Catholic family, and you may recall I'm Jewish. Get my anxiety?"

"Oh yeah, I get it. Tell me more."

"Well, she grew up in Southie and my picture of Southie is that it's homogeneous, pretty much. A lot of stories about attitudes towards anyone not Irish Catholic. I could be wrong, but that's on my mind.

"Cathy and I, well, we're in love. I haven't proposed, but I'm planning to. But we have these sensitive religious and ethnic differences. We don't feel them so much, but we're worried both sets of parents may have serious reservations. And I'm not exactly a regular kind of guy, with my paralysis. So, any advice how to handle this meeting with her parents?"

Susan took in a deep breath, considered what Ben had said, and replied after a few moments.

"Ben, best wishes on your romance. That's great news, I'm so glad for you.

"Here are a few things that come to mind. First, talk with Cathy. Ask her to describe her parents, what they're like, their temperaments, their world view, and what she thinks their response will be. She's known them all her life. And surely, she's talked with them about this, so have her fill you in on her expectations.

"Secondly, have your own agenda before you go. What do you hope to get out of this meeting? Her parents' attitudes about all kinds of things. Have a mental list of non-controversial topics you can fall back on when silence prevails -- sports, movies, books and so on. Avoid getting into religion or politics, always touchy areas. Talk about Cathy's siblings. Talk about her dad's work. Find out about her mother's interests and what she does each day. People always like to talk about themselves, so focus as much as possible on them. Respond to their questions about you and your goals in life. And above all, be yourself. You're a special person."

That last comment brought a lump to his throat. He swallowed, and said,

"Those ideas are just the framework I needed. Thanks. Can I get back to you, either before or after the meeting, for further advice?"

"Sure. I'm glad you called. It's good to hear from you and even better to hear of your life plans with Cathy. Keep me posted."

Why didn't I think to ask Cathy those questions? I guess when you're in the thick of solving problems, the things right in front of your face don't occur to you.

He was on duty that evening, so he called Cathy the following night. He got right to the point. "Can you tell me some basic stuff about your parents? You know, I don't even know their first names, what they enjoy doing, hobbies, sports interests, that kind of thing," he asked, his voice rising a bit with anxiety. "And are they real serious, observant Catholics? Democrats or Republicans? How is your relationship with them? Things I should avoid discussing with them? Should I bring a gift?"

Cathy chuckled as she heard Ben's nervous questions.

"Let's start with their first names: John and Meg. Dad goes as 'Jack.' Meg is short for Megan. They're around fifty, both born and raised in Southie. Childhood sweethearts. Mom goes to mass faithfully every week, usually unaccompanied by Dad, who gets impatient with what he calls 'churchy things.'

"They're both Democrats, but not exactly liberal. Neither would ever vote Republican, not so much because of any political ideology, but because in Southie you just don't vote for Republicans."

"Have you talked to them about me?"

"Of course. They know about your disability; they know you're Jewish. They know you're from a wealthy Chestnut Hill family. And that your dad is a jeweler."

"And what do they say about those first two things?"

"They wonder about both. They worry about me in a caretaker role since they don't see me as a caretaker. Neither do I, but then I don't consider myself as your caretaker anyway. You can do most things you need to, and what you can't do, you figure out a way to get it done. They do know I'm madly, deeply in love with you."

Ben felt a warm tingle when he heard this. "Do they know their good Catholic daughter is living in sin with me?"

"Good heavens, no! Even I have my limit when it comes to sharing with my parents." After switching the phone to her other ear, she said, "Their attitude about your being a Jew is hard for me to know. They say all the right things, like 'some of my best friends are Jewish.' Neither of them has ever been in a synagogue nor participated in a Passover celebration. For that matter, neither have I."

"Well, since my Bar Mitzvah, I've hardly set foot inside a temple either," Ben said. "I've been schooled in Hebrew beliefs, but I'm not devout. I guess I could be called a 'cafeteria Jew' like Catholics who don't buy the whole package. I am sensitive, though, to anything that smacks of anti-Semitism, just as I am upset with racism, and other isms that go against common decency.

"Going on," Cathy said, "Dad is an electrician, has his own company, along with two of my brothers. They work all over Boston. You may have seen his signs 'Kelly and Sons,' and his slogan, 'We'll light up your life.' Corny, but effective. Outside of work, everyone in the whole family is an avid Red Sox and Bruins fan. Even Mom."

"That's good to know. I love the Sox. Not so much hockey. I'm also a Celtics fan. But you already knew that."

"Oh, forgot basketball. They love Red Auerbach, Cousy, Sharman and McCauley. I do too."

"Well, this helps a lot. Talking sports is usually a safe topic. Unless, of course, you're a Yankees fan," Ben said. "Also, I'll studiously avoid sensitive issues."

"They will, too. They'll be on their best behavior." Sensing they were done with this topic, at least for now, she went on. "Can we get together this weekend?"

"For sure. I'm off from Friday night until Monday morning. One of the few times I have a whole weekend off."

"How'd you work that?"

"Changing services over the weekend. It just works out that way."

"Which night do you want to spend with me?"

"Every night. But how about Friday and Saturday night, then I'll go home and spend most of Sunday with my folks. They kinda miss me, and I miss them, too. Besides, it's easier to be at home the night before I start the week on Monday."

"Sounds good. I get home around 5:00 on Friday. Come when you can."

Their weekend together was glorious. They ate well, enjoyed the sunshine and moving around Jamaica Pond, drank South African pinot noir at all their meals, made love often and exquisitely, and slept late. Ben envied the dog walking couples and looked forward to the day when he could once more have a Lab like Slocum.

Chapter 29

Salk Vaccine

This month, Ben was on the hematology/oncology service. He'd heard from other interns that caring for kids who were dying from leukemia and other tumors was the most depressing rotation of the internship. It was a wonder to him, then, that many of his colleagues would ultimately choose to go further into that field. Each year fellowships in hematology/oncology filled early. *Had to be the challenge of finding a cure for cancer,* he thought.

After he'd been on the service a couple of weeks, Ben marveled at how kids, despite being very sick, were upbeat in their acceptance of their plight. He initially thought it was childlike naivete about their prognosis that allowed them to stay positive. He realized, though, as he spent more time on the ward, that other reasons were responsible: the love of their families and the love of the medical team that made this potentially depressing situation more acceptable than rational thought would suggest.

Monday morning, Ben got there early to get acquainted with some of the patients before rounds began. He stopped first at Gordon Walter's bed.

Gordon, a 16-year-old boy, was a second-string quarterback on the varsity football team. He fell while practicing with his mates. "It just gave way on me," he'd said of his right leg when he came to the hospital. "It didn't hurt before I fell, but it sure did later," he told the doctors.

He'd fractured his femur and X-rays showed not only a fracture but also a tumor, establishing this break as a pathological fracture, pathology in this case being an osteosarcoma. This malignant tumor was particularly difficult to treat, when seen in an extremity, usually requiring amputation above the tumor and a meticulous examination of other regions of the body for possible metastatic disease. Gordon now was ten days post-surgery and now learning how to attach his prosthesis to what was left of his leg.

Ben wheeled up to his bedside and began a conversation with him.

"Hello, Gordon. How goes it today?"

"Well, okay, I guess. Sorry, who are you?"

"I'm Ben, new intern on the floor. Just starting this rotation. Tell me why you're here."

"They operated and took my leg off above the knee about ten days ago. Had to do that to get rid of the tumor. Still feeling the leg is there. The other doctors told me this is common, called 'phantom limb.' Don't like it much, I can tell you."

"How's the new prosthesis?" Ben said, noticing it on the bed.

"Still tender around the top part where it attaches to my thigh, but I guess I'll have to get used to that. Hard to put any weight on it." His gaze fixed intently on Ben's wheelchair.

"You're wondering why I'm in this wheelchair. It's because of polio. It took me a while to get used to it but now I'm okay with it. I figured I had no choice."

"When did that happen?"

"A couple of years ago. I was 23 and in medical school. Took care of a kiddo with polio and probably picked it up from him."

"Boy, sure glad I never got polio. That disease scares me, scares everyone. What I got is bad enough. But you made it through school, and here you are, a doctor. That's really something."

"I'm proud of all the people who cared for me -- my parents, all the doctors, nurses and others who kept me going when I was down. It just goes to show we all must play the hand we're dealt. You seem to be doing that. Keep up the good work."

Ben, for the first time, began to see his disability as a peculiar advantage as he took care of young patients with challenging medical problems of their own. They could identify with him as someone who had been sick but now was back doing his work. Seeing him could be a source of hope as they battled their way back from illness.

He moved on to see Julie, a 4-year-old girl, sleeping with an intravenous line carrying a blood transfusion into her frail body. She had bruises mottling her arms. Ben picked up her chart from the end of the bed. Her diagnosis was acute lymphoblastic leukemia, the most common cancer in this age group. He saw that her red blood cell count indicated profound anemia and part of the blood clotting mechanism, the platelets, were low, accounting for her bruises. He didn't want to wake her up, and rounds were about to start, so he joined the group, introducing himself to each of the five in the group.

Together, they first saw Mitchell, an 18-year-old boy, who had Hodgkin disease for which there was currently no successful treatment. He was on an experimental drug, but it hadn't helped. The next patient was a diagnostic dilemma. She was from Guatemala and had anemia of unknown origin. Tests had ruled out all the usual suspects. Now the team was chasing down rare causes, but so far there were no diagnostic entities that fit her case. This would be called a fascinoma, a term the medical team used for unsolved and interesting illnesses.

Ben continued to be impressed with the range of diseases he was seeing. Dr. Friedman was right -- pediatrics was distinct from internal medicine. Children were not little adults. He hadn't yet encountered the assortment of infectious diseases most commonly seen in the pediatric general wards, ranging from streptococcal infections and its residua, glomerulonephritis and rheumatic fever; poliomyelitis, ear infections, sepsis, measles, mumps, chickenpox, hepatitis, parasitic diseases, Rocky Mountain Spotted fever, and fungus infections, like histoplasmosis and coccidiomycosis. Asthma was still another problem, often affecting inner-city poor kids. Some physicians blamed it on allergies to house dust, others blamed air pollutions, still others thought it was due to mold. Ben was immersed in a wealth of learning.

"Ben, have you heard the good news?" Adam asked.

"What good news? I've been so inundated with patients and scut work I haven't lifted my head up."

"The Salk vaccine field trials evaluations were successful. They claim a 60-80% effectiveness for all three strains of polio. The Secretary of Health Education and Welfare endorsed the National Foundation for Infantile Paralysis' recommendation to license the Salk vaccine. So, a vaccine for polio is now a reality."

Ben sighed. "I'm so glad it's finally done. I've been following the drama of the two camps who've been jousting over which kind of vaccine is best, the killed one of Salk's lab or the live attenuated one from Sabin's lab. It's been like the Yankees and the Red Sox rivalry. Salk versus Sabin. Looks like Salk won out. Right?"

"Yes, at least for now. Sabin is still beating the drum for a live vaccine since he claims that it not only protects the kids that get the vaccine but has a herd immunity effect by spreading the live attenuated virus in the community.

"The real winners in this professional argument, though, are the kids and their families," Adam said. "Jonas Salk has endured his share of bad press because of, I guess, his sort of a celebrity status and an abundant amount of his own hubris. But he was quoted, in answer to a reporter's question about who owned the patent on the vaccine, said, "Well, the people, I would say. There is no patent. Could you patent the sun?"

"That's a quote for the ages," Ben said. "No matter what has been said about him, that is true altruism. No other way to say it."

~~~

Days turned into weeks, and the time to meet Cathy's parents was approaching. Ben had been so overwhelmed with the demands of internship that he'd talked to Cathy only three times in the past couple of weeks. After admitting patients all day and then relaying the status of patients to the intern covering the pediatric service for the night, he'd go home and fall into bed, asleep as soon as he pulled the covers over
~~~

his body. On this night, though, before he fell into the arms of Morpheus, he called Cathy.

"Hi Cath. We still on for this Sunday to meet your folks?" She could tell how fatigued he was by the weakness of his voice.

"Absolutely. They're eager to meet you. Pick me up around eleven and we'll have plenty of time to get there and get into the house. They suggested we go into the driveway to the back door since the front door is up about five stairs and the back door is on flat ground."

"Okay. I'm gonna sign off. I'm wiped out. Goodnight. I love you."

"Love you too. See you Sunday."

Sunday came and Ben picked Cathy up and headed to Southie. They arrived in front of the house and Ben took note of the architecture, the color, and the setting. It was a Victorian, with dentate molding around the joints at the top of clapboards, curlicue decorations on the side panels, bay windows dominating the front exterior wall, a porch with five steps ascending to a small, enclosed porch with sculptured balustrades supporting the railings. A great oak door featuring two bull's eye windows across the top had an antique knob that looked that it would take a weightlifting athlete to operate it. Ben was glad they were going in the back door.

Ben parked the Suburban in an open area, allowing for him to get out, do his routine with braces and crutches, unload the chair, and roll into the house on a level surface from the driveway. Once inside, they shed their coats and proceeded into the dining room, where Jack and Meg welcomed them warmly.

"So glad to get to meet you finally, Ben. Cathy has told us all about you. How are you?" Meg said with Jack standing and smiling at her side.

"I'm glad for the chance to get acquainted," he said, hoping his greeting was not too perfunctory. He felt awkward and looked to Cathy for guidance. She obliged him by saying,

"Where would you like us to congregate?"

"Let's go into the front room," Meg answered. She was a trim 58-year-old brunette, an older version of Cathy. Jack had white hair and plenty of it, a face with deep lines like parentheses around his mouth. He stood six feet tall and could have been an ad for middle age fitness.

Their capacious living room was decorated with period furniture dating from early in the 20th century. Cathy sat on a loveseat with a carved wooden frame and a needlepoint fabric, Ben stayed in his wheelchair. A grand piano graced the bay that looked out through a large, curved window onto the street. Meg sat on her favorite wing chair. Jack took drink orders.

"Just a coke for me," Ben said. He knew if he drank any alcohol, he'd fall asleep.

Cathy and Meg both asked for tea, with lemon and sugar.

Jack came back with the drinks, and they began a predictable but necessary script.

"Tell us a little bit about yourself, Ben," Meg said.

"Well, I grew up in Chestnut Hill, went to school in Brookline, then to Channing University and Channing Medical School. Now I'm at Suffolk County Hospital for my internship."

"Like it there?" Jack asked.

"Love it. I'm learning so much."

"I have a soft place in my heart for Suffolk County Hospital," Jack said. "I was born there as were most of my family. I knew Mary Flannigan's son as I was growing up. Her father was Mayor, you know, and that's how the Pediatric Building came to be named the Mary Flannigan Building."

"Yeah, that history was described to us when we all started our internship. Quite a family."

"So, what do you plan on doing when you finish training?" Jack asked.

"I hope to stay on as faculty there. I'd like to teach, do some clinical research. I think I can make my contribution best that way. Also, with my disability it seems like the best path for me."

Ben deliberately opened the discussion about his paralysis, so it could be disposed of early. He wanted to know about their attitudes around Cathy's involvement with a "crippled man." He told them about his polio and subsequent rehabilitation and retraining for daily living.

"You got it from a patient, right? That's what Cathy told us," Jack said.

"Yes. Timmy was his name. He died after being in an iron lung for some time. I knew him well and loved him like he was my own child. I was devastated. He was such a good kid."

"That must have been awful for you," Meg said. She looked at Jack and said, "We have friends who had a child who got polio. They were terrified. His only paralysis was in his face. He has a crooked smile, but that's all."

"Yes, it was tough seeing Timmy go through that. We thought he would throw off the need for the lung, but it never happened. He got pneumonia from a different germ altogether. It's difficult keeping infections away from immobilized patients. That's what killed him.

"But paralysis occurs in only a small percentage of those who get polio. That could change in future epidemics, though. The good news, you've probably heard, is that a vaccine has been developed in Pittsburgh. Dr. Jonas Salk worked on that with his team. What a breakthrough, when all kids everywhere will be immunized and protected from getting polio. Like smallpox, diphtheria, whooping cough, and tetanus."

Ben hoped that by opening this door to discussing his disability they could face it head-on, but what he'd said succeeded only in casting a pall over further dialogue. A few moments ticked by in silence and then Meg said, "Anyone hungry?"

Ben grinned, both disappointed and relieved that no more would be said now about his paralysis, nodded his head, and said, "Three guesses!" Everyone laughed and they went to the dining room. Ben moved his chair into a space they'd created on one side of the table. Meg brought out roast chicken, spinach, and mashed potatoes with gravy.

"I understand you run an electrical company," Ben said to Jack, doing what Susan suggested.

"Right. Been wiring people's houses since I was 20. It's interesting work. I meet all kinds of people, get to hear about their lives and see how they live. I enjoy it."

"And your boys are in it with you?"

"Yeah. They joined me after they got their education in the Voc/Tech school in Dorchester. They can do things I never knew how to do, so it works out."

"Ben, tell them about your car, how it's equipped with special levers to allow you to drive," Cathy said. "It works very well. He's a good driver."

"Maybe after dinner I can show it to you," he offered.

"I'd really like to see that," Jack said.

"Me too," Meg added.

After dinner they all went out to the Suburban. Ben showed them the DriveMaster lever system and his routine for moving from the driver's seat to the rear of the car and retrieving his chair.

"Quite a system you have," Jack said, clearly impressed. "I've never seen that DriveMaster before. You feel comfortable driving with it?"

"Very comfortable now. It took some getting used to at first. But now I'm able to do most everything I want."

"And I feel perfectly safe driving with him," Cathy said. "The first time, I was nervous as hell. But now I see he's got complete control."

Back in the living room they all relaxed, now having become somewhat acquainted with one another. They talked about Jack's work, Cathy's interests in public health, Meg's book group and her painting classes, Ben's experiences at the hospital, and, of course, the Red Sox. By the end of the visit, Ben felt the first visit with Cathy's parents went well, like Cathy's visit with his parents. Future visits were sure to raise issues they would have to address, but for now, all was well.

Chapter 30

No Longer an Intern, July 1954

As the month of June concluded, so did the so-called "year of purgatory." Internship, seemingly an eternity, was mercifully over and every other night on-duty was history. Now that obligation would be every third night, which seemed almost like vacation as Ben moved up to his first year of residency. His first rotation was on general pediatrics where most cases were admitted and stayed unless they required specialized attention.

He felt more at home now, seasoned during internship, eager to narrow his focus on areas that mattered most to him. The field of community pediatrics, although not even yet named as such, was crystallizing in his mind. He recalled Uncle Abraham's advice to him. "The main thing you need is desire and curiosity. The other thing you need is a sense of duty. A sense of community, like we're all in this together.

Being a practicing doctor is a calling. It's not just a job or a way to make a living. It's a sense that you must do this. Sort of a religious experience. You just know.

It's that voice in your head that tells you what's right and wrong, what you should do. I don't know where it comes from. Some people believe it's from God, others believe it's from your family or community or something else."

Rounds began with a new cadre of residents and interns. Today, the clinical team was standing at the bed of a tiny girl, born unexpectedly four weeks before, at home without benefit of a midwife or a physical exam of the newborn baby, and brought to the hospital during the night by ambulance.

"Her breathing was shallow and rapid, respiratory rate 60 per minute," the neophyte admitting intern reported, as the papers in his hand trembled. "Her heart rate was 150, X-rays showed an enlarged heart. When I listened to her heart, I was stunned. Her heart murmur was the loudest I've ever heard. I consulted the cardiology fellow, and as soon as he listened, suspected a ventricular septal defect." Dr. Jenkins, the preceptor, turned to the medical students and quizzed them: "What is a ventricular septal defect?" The students looked at each other and one said, "A hole in the wall separating two of the pumping chambers of the heart, the two ventricles."

"So, why is that bad?"

"The left ventricle shunts blood to the right ventricle instead of pumping all of it out to the main arteries going to the body," the student replied. "At this early age, the resistance in the lungs is greater than it is later, and pulmonary hypertension results."

"And then what happens?"

"The heart tries to overcome that by beating faster and gradually the heart enlarges, then fails to do its job."

"Very good. So, what is the clinical plan?" he asked, turning back to the Intern.

"The cardiac surgeons are coming to see the baby," the Intern said. I hope they get on it right away. She doesn't look good at all."

"Stay here with the baby until the surgeons arrive," Dr. Jenkins told the intern, still unnerved by this very serious case, the first patient of his internship. "We're going to move along and complete our rounds. Call us immediately if things start tanking." The intern's eyes darted around looking for help, but knew he had no choice but to do as he was told.

The team proceeded down the line of beds, all with crying children. One had aseptic meningitis and was being watched carefully after bacterial meningitis had been ruled out by negative bacteriologic cultures; another child was suffering joint pains from juvenile rheumatoid arthritis. There was a spirited discussion about the dose of steroids to be used.

"What are the downsides of using steroids?" Jenkins asked.

"Using steroids can depress the body's natural production of steroids by the adrenal gland," one of the medical students said.

"Right." Turning to the other new intern, he said, "Tell us about this child with this rash."

"It's all over his body. He's really miserable."

"What is the differential diagnosis?" Dr. Jenkins asked, referring to the exercise of listing all the possibilities when confronted with a diagnostic dilemma.

"Could be a whole lot of things," the intern said.

"That's not an answer. What things?"

"Well," the intern stammered, embarrassed. "Measles, I guess, and other viral rashes."

"How about scarlet fever? Meningococcemia? Roseola? You better go study Nelson's textbook and learn more about exanthems. This could be quite serious."

Jenkins turned to Ben and asked about the boy.

"Mother said she picked a small black 'thing' off his waistband, but she didn't bring it to the hospital, so our assumption was that it was a dog tick. The working diagnosis is Rocky Mountain spotted fever while we wait for lab studies to return."

By the time they finished rounds, the cardiac surgeons had transferred the baby with congestive heart failure to their surgical suite, doing diagnostic testing to decide about surgical intervention. Their concern matched that of the intern and nurses who had watched her.

Ben rolled out to the corridor looking for Adam on the hematology/oncology ward down the hall. He spotted him and asked if he could join him for lunch.

"I have to draw some blood, but I'll meet you at Billy's, okay? Don't take the route you did the last time," he laughed. "I could be too late this time." Ben smiled wryly, not very amused since that frightening experience still lingered in his thoughts and had awakened him from sleep. "Should I order for you?"

"Yeah, get me the gyro and chips," he said.

Ben waited for Adam at their usual table. He arrived fifteen minutes later with a scowl.

"What's up?" Ben asked.

"One of my patients, an Irish teenager, gave me a hard time with his racist attitude. Pissed me off."

"What did he say?"

"He looked at me and said, 'Boy, you sure you know what to do?' as I was drawing his blood."

"What did you do?"

"I pretended to ignore him. I got into his vein perfectly. I wasn't gonna give him the satisfaction of knowing he got under my skin. My black skin, that is."

"Do you think we'll ever have a color-blind world?" Ben asked, shaking his head.

"Fat chance. I thought Maryland was bad. But it doesn't matter where you go if you're not white. There are racists everywhere. I can't go jogging without some white jerk looking at me with fear on his face -- or hatred -- as though I'm gonna attack him. Chances are more likely that he'll attack me."

Ben didn't know how to respond. He was tempted to bring up anti-Semitism, but decided they were not completely comparable, and besides, it wouldn't help Adam to hear about another tribe's problems when he was trying to work out his own. So, he said, "I got your gyro," indicating the package on the table. "I didn't know what you wanted to drink."

"Oh, I'll get that. Thanks. What's the toll?"

"Forget it. Pay for lunch tomorrow. We can go someplace expensive," he laughed. Looking directly at Adam, he said, "Aside from that bad experience, how's Heme/Onc looking on your first day?"

"A lot better as a resident than an intern," Adam said. "But I don't think that's the field I want to spend my life in. I want to do general pediatrics in an underserved community."

"Maybe you and I ought to try to stay here, get on faculty. I'm thinking about a new field I'm calling 'community pediatrics.' Don't ask me exactly what that is yet. Residency training is mainly hospital-based, you know, real sick kids, but most pediatric patients never get admitted, are sick at home, or have things that need to be taken care of in outpatient clinics. Things like growth or developmental problems, or psychological issues. I'm also interested in kids with disabilities. Not hard to see why I'm interested in that.

But I want to see health care given, like you, where it's most needed. And that means not only health care, but helping these populations with other things they need, like better housing, job training, schools, even legal advice. You know, some doctors like going to third world places to care for those populations. I think that would be difficult for me in a wheelchair, and besides, there's so much need right here in this country."

"Some people might think you're a socialist or something with those ideas. Be careful. I agree with you about the need, but you could run into trouble with your 'save the world' ideas that threaten the old status quo."

"I'm ready to fight for these things if it comes to that. I love this country, but I see things that scream to be changed."

"You sound like my dad preacher, brother Ben! You'll have to meet him someday. You'd get along well."

"I'd like that. If your folks ever come to Boston, they can stay at our house. By the way, we need to have you over for dinner, meet my folks, and meet Cathy.

"You have a girl friend?"

"Not here, but at home. She's in a nursing school in Baltimore."

"Well, she and your parents could all come together!"

"I'll work on it. That'd be great."

When Ben got home that night, he ran this idea by his parents.

"Maybe we could all go to a Red Sox game, come back here for dinner," Sophie said. "Have any idea when his parents could come?"

"I think we should go ahead and schedule a time for Adam to come by himself," Jacob said, "go to a ballgame, back here for dinner, plan for his parents and girlfriend to come later. That visit is more complicated."

"Yeah, agree with that," Ben said. "You know, I've wondered about going to a Red Sox game, whether I could handle Fenway Park. But if you and Adam were there, I think I could manage. Let's pick a date. Whaddya think, Dad?" turning to Jacob.

"I know a guy at the Red Sox ticket office. When we set a date, I'll talk to him. Let's do it. Sounds terrific."

~~~

The next day on the wards several new admissions got the team's attention. A three-year-old girl came in seizing. She was treated successfully in the emergency room with intravenous phenobarbital, but she was still agitated and moaning in apparent pain, so she was admitted. Her mother said she'd been listless, had vomited several times before coming to the hospital, and seemed very irritable. They did X-rays of her abdomen because of her pain and vomiting. These showed spotty shadows in many areas of the gut. The
~~~

radiologist said these looked like they were radio-opaque lead. The lab results confirmed wildly elevated lead levels in her blood. It was clear this was lead poisoning.

"This seems to be increasing in incidence," Ben told the team. "What can we do about it?"

"Educate parents to be on the lookout for pica in their kids," one student said.

"Do you all know what pica is?" Ben asked, looking around at the medical students.

Glances all around, until one of them said, "I think it means eating non-food objects."

"Right! Good for you. Telling parents about pica is important. What else?" Ben asked.

"Have parents recognize early symptoms and bring their kids in," another said.

"Yes. There's more, though."

The students and intern looked at each other. *"What's he after?"* they wondered.

"When we have a child with an infection, what do we look for?" Ben asked, teaching by analogy.

"The organism responsible for the infection?" a student said cautiously.

"Right! So, what's responsible for lead poisoning?"

"Duh, lead," a wise guy student said with a smirk.

"And where do these kids get lead?" Ben said, ignoring the sarcasm.

"Eating peeling paint, it seems, containing lead."

"Correct again. So, what should we be doing?"

"Getting the lead out," Mr. Wise Guy said, laughing. "Of their environment,"

"What does that mean?" Ben said, still ignoring this feeble attempt at humor by Mr. Wise Guy.

"Finding and eliminating the lead paint in houses before the kids can eat the paint chips," Mr. Wise Guy said, this time in a serious tone.

"Will that be an easy fix?" Ben asked rhetorically. "I'll answer that for you. Not at all. Is that our job? To find and eliminate lead paint in all the housing that has it?"

"The city Health Department should be doing that," another student offered. "Not really a doctor's job."

"I'd like to have you all think more about that. Is it really not the doctor's job? We can discuss it more tomorrow. But now we need to get going to see the other patients," Ben said.

The next patient they saw had diarrhea. "In these cases," Ben said, "the most pressing problem is dehydration. Starting intravenous solutions, making sure the balance of electrolytes matches the patient's age and size, is critical. So, cases of diarrhea require initial blood levels of sodium and potassium to calculate how much of those should be given."

It was tricky to find veins for intravenous infusions in these little people, but Ben was good at getting needles into tiny veins. To calculate the right mix of sodium and potassium he taught the interns a "secret" formula he remembered from one of his teachers in medical school.

Ben loved teaching medical students and interns. "What are the usual causes of diarrhea?" he asked them. "Shigella, salmonella, and E. coli," one student said.

"Yeah, those are common bacterial causes," Ben said. "But most cases are not from bacteria but viruses, particularly rotavirus. However, you still need to get bacterial cultures of the stools, but aware that most will be negative."

Ben was in his element, teaching and exchanging ideas with other students of medicine. He was gripped by a feeling, an almost palpable spiritual experience, a metamorphosis. Uncle Abraham's words kept returning to him: medicine was a calling, a transcendent becoming. He was changing from Ben Levinson, a person, to Benjamin Nathan Levinson, the Physician. He felt this was what he was meant to be.

Chapter 31

Take Me Out to the Ballgame

Ben stopped Adam in the hall. "How 'bout a Red Sox game and dinner with Cathy and my folks? Interested?"

"Hell yes! Love to meet your parents -- and Cathy. And free home-cooked dinners are always welcome! Attending a Red Sox game might be another matter," Adam said, smiling broadly. "I can't root for the Sox, you know, if they play the Orioles. I'd have to root for my O's."

Turning serious, he said "My other problem is with Fenway. I could meet some hostility. It's got a reputation for not welcoming people my color. But I've never been there, so I have no firsthand experience."

"I didn't know that about Fenway," Ben said, reminded once more of his naivete about racism in Boston. "Let's go anyway. We'll just ignore any drunk rednecks in the stands."

"Yeah, I'd like to go. Fenway Park! 'A little bandbox' of a baseball park," Adam said. "This could be an important lesson for us about racism in Boston.

I'll be interested to see your take. Pay attention to little knowing glances between people, raised eyebrows and behind-cupped-hand comments."

"I'll watch," Ben said, feeling somewhat uncomfortable about his friend's suspicious attitude. "I hope you're wrong. Wish I could say I'll protect you like you did when those two kids threatened me. But I'm not exactly the kind of guy who inspires fear," he added with a rueful smile. "So, it sounds like a plan," Ben said, avoiding further discussion. "Give me some dates when you're off-duty, I'll match them with times that my folks, Cathy and I can go. We'll set it up. I'll try to find a date when the Red Sox play the Yankees. That way we can all cheer for the Sox."

Ben called Sophie, Jacob and Cathy about his invitation to Adam and asked for their availability and then said, "Dad, can you order the tickets?"

"Sure. Five tickets. I'll wait for the date."

They met at the Levinson's house on Sunday, August 15, and Jacob drove to Fenway, dropping all of them off at the main gate. Adam helped Ben negotiate the way to their seats. Jacob got box seats behind first base and the Red Sox dugout. They could hear the chatter in the dugout and see the players' faces as they moved in and out of the dugout during the game.

"Your dad did an amazing job getting these great seats," Adam told Ben when they'd gotten settled. "I hope he doesn't have trouble finding parking."

"Don't worry, he's got a lot of connections around here. He'll have no trouble. He's sold jewelry to guys on the team and their wives and a lot of the people who have businesses around the ballpark. He even knows the owner of the team. No problem," Ben said proudly.

Jacob strolled in about ten minutes later with a smile on his face and sat next to Sophie, just behind Adam, Ben, and Cathy.

"Whadda guy!" Cathy beamed at Jacob. "Terrific seats, Thanks!" Jacob smiled back in his usual reticent manner, acknowledging the gratitude.

It wasn't long before it was clear this was not going to be a good day for the Mudville nine. The Yankees scored eight runs in the visitor's first half-inning before most people were even in their seats and six more in the later innings. The Sox got nine runs scattered over the balance of play with Jimmy Piersall leading the way with three hits, but the die was cast in that first inning. The final score was 14-9, in favor of the Yankees in this slugfest. The fans, although disappointed with the loss, enjoyed the game with all the action.

"Well, that was not what we'd hoped for, but what a game!" Ben said to Adam.

"So much fun to be here, after all my angst and fears. I can't wait to tell my folks about it. Thanks to your family for making this happen," Adam said.

Ben had no need to find a bathroom so that challenge was averted. He did notice occasional long stares at Adam from some fans near their seats, but the afternoon passed with no overt signs of disapproval to lessen the afternoon's enjoyment by the Levinsons' entourage. They went home for dinner with a feeling of pure pleasure.

"Hamburgers or hot dogs?" Jacob asked everyone when they got back at the Levinson house. "Cooked to perfection by me on the grill. A beautiful summer's day even though we lost the game. The good news—we can eat outside on the deck!"

Their deck was adjacent to a neatly trimmed lawn surrounded by a mix of tall oak and hemlock trees. Flower beds in full bloom and overflowing with colors dotted the periphery of the yard. When the food was ready, Sophie brought greens and her famous German potato salad, sprinkled with tarragon, parsley, and poppy seeds.

"What did the Orioles do today?" Ben asked Adam.

"I just checked. Lost too," he said. "Not a good day for our teams. But at least we have a better record than the hapless Red Sox," he teased.

"Season's not over, buddy," Ben said, rising to the bait. "It's a long season and anything can happen."

"Yeah, and pigs fly sometimes, right?"

"We'll see when the Orioles play the Sox next time. But you're not invited to that game 'cause you'll be rooting for the wrong team."

The banter went on until Sophie admonished, "Listen you two, if you don't stop you can't have my potato salad. Or dessert."

"He started it," Ben said, reverting to adolescent repartee, but with a smile.

"Okay, I did, but it's not a fair fight. You got your mother on your side," Adam laughed.

Cathy smiled at all this. "Feels just like home," she said. "Just like the script my brothers follow after a game. One is a Yankees fan, so you can imagine what that's like."

"I see why you moved out," Ben said with a big grin. "And so glad you did!"

"So, where do you live Cathy?" Adam asked.

"J.P. Over a restaurant. I love it. Smells delicious all the time."

"Where do you live, Adam?" Jacob asked.

"An apartment in the high rise near the hospital. Owned by the hospital. Interns and residents get a big break on rent. Gym and swimming pool downstairs. And a parking garage. Don't have a car, so I don't need that. Lots of hospital staff park there."

"Do you like the hospital?" Sophie asked, shading her eyes against the sun. Ben worried she might express her critical view of Suffolk County Hospital.

"It's so reminiscent of Baltimore City that I immediately fell in love with the place. I feel right at home there."

"Ben told us your father is a minister. Right?" Sophie asked.

"Yeah, in an AME church in Cambridge, Maryland."

"Better explain what AME is," Ben said.

"African Methodist Episcopalian." He told them what he'd told Ben before.

"What does your mother do?" Sophie inquired.

"She's a nurse, works with the VNA on the eastern shore," Adam said. "She knows a lot about sickle cell anemia since my younger brother has it. Her nursing job and my brother's illness both played parts in my wanting to be a doctor."

"Do you think we can get your family to visit us?" Sophie said.

"I'll ask them. It's difficult juggling Dad's responsibilities with the congregation, Mom's schedule, and my brother's condition. We never know when he's gonna have a problem. But I'll talk to them about it. Nice you asked."

"Could we get your girlfriend to come up and visit?" Ben asked.

"That's probably easier. I'll talk to her. She's a social worker with a county agency. She'd probably welcome a break. She deals with a lot of unhappiness."

"Let's get this done before winter makes it difficult," Jacob said. "What's your girlfriend's name?"

"Sarah."

"Would she be more likely to come if I sent a personal invitation?" Sophie said.

"Yes, she'd be more likely to come if she got an invitation from you. That'd be great."

"Just so she's not an Orioles fan," Ben laughed.

"She's not even a baseball fan," Adam said. "Says it's a boring game."

"Well, let's call the whole thing off!" Ben said. "If she can't appreciate the most wonderful sporting contest there is, what would we have to talk about?"

"Maybe art, or music, travel, or nature?" Cathy dove into the conversation, laughing. "You guys are so predictable."

"Okay, okay. I'm just joking," Ben said.

They finished their meal and Sophie brought out Ben's favorite mixed berry pie with ice cream. Afterwards, Ben took Adam back to the hospital and Cathy to her apartment. After parking, he recruited the friendly waiters at the restaurant to get him up to Cathy's apartment where he spent the night.

"Cathy, I have an important question to ask," Ben said.

She looked at him, wondering what he was about to ask. There were so many issues in their young lives: their individual career trajectories; Ben's disability, parents with disparate backgrounds, religions, and belief systems; racial problems in Boston and the country beyond. So many unsettled problems facing everyone in this confusing maelstrom called contemporary life.

"What?"

"Will you marry me?"

The vacant space this quiet held was immense. An eternity might have passed before she answered. But finally, she said, "Yes, I will. Gladly. I love you with all my heart and soul and have since I first saw you. Hold me. Tight."

Ben held her and he brushed tears away as the relief of joy spread throughout his chest. His breathing calmed him. He turned her head toward his face and kissed hers face, her lips, her eyes, her cheeks, her neck and down to her breasts. They were transported.

When they awoke, they looked at one another with a new understanding, one that lifted them both from an ordinary day to one filled with expectation and hope.

Chapter 32

Sophie, Meg, Jacob, and Jack

Ben and Cathy called both of their parents the next day.

"We're getting married. Can we talk?"

Sophie looked at Jacob after they ended the call.

"Are you surprised?"

"No. Are you?"

"Hardly. Now what?"

"I think we have to recognize that we, as Reform Jews, need to acknowledge certain things," Jacob said. "First, we haven't raised Ben in the Orthodox tradition. Sure, he had a Bar Mitzvah, but we've never been regulars at synagogue. So, his intention to marry outside of the Jewish community shouldn't come to us as a surprise."

"But, after all that Jews have gone through," Sophie said, "I feel an allegiance to our people. If we don't maintain that, what will happen to us all?"

"It reminds me of that show in the 20's," Jacob said. "Remember? Called Abie's Irish Rose? An Irish

Catholic and an American Jew marry over the objections of both sets of parents."

"I never saw it. Wasn't that before we came to America? But I did hear about it. It got terrible critical reviews as I recall."

"But it was wildly popular. That story concludes with the parents all finally accepting the marriage."

"I don't know," Sophie lamented. "Maybe we should have stayed closer to our heritage and taught Benji more about Judaism. Maybe then he wouldn't have considered marrying outside."

"Too late now. I think most Reform Jews will gradually stop resisting Jews marrying non-Jews."

"There'll always be those who will resist. How many we don't know. But as long as there are some, they'll always shun those who marry outside. Shicksas will always be shut out. I like Cathy and feel bad that she might suffer that kind of discrimination. But it's the truth. She won't be accepted by some, and the ones who don't accept her may be very vocal and powerful."

"All that doesn't mean much when it comes to what we do. Ben has decided. Cathy has too. The way I see it is that we either accommodate to it or," Jacob grabbed Sophie's hand as he continued, "we lose Ben and the children they'll have. Our grandchildren."

Sophie looked for tissues to dry her eyes. She was reliving the day when she had the operation that made it impossible to have any babies after Ben. Now she pondered an unthinkable potential further, additional loss, of grandchildren.

"I need time. I need advice from someone. I don't know. Everyone we know will have a strong opinion. I have to think this through." Looking at Jacob through her tears, she murmured, "It sounds like you've made up your mind. Your opinion is important, Jacob. But it's not, you know, binding upon me. Give me some time."

"Of course, Sophie. I'll tell Ben we need time to think."

In South Boston, Jack and Meg also got the news with ambivalence.

"She was always headstrong, you know. Once she got an idea, she wouldn't change her mind," Meg said to Jack. "Stubborn little girl. Stubborn adolescent. Now a stubborn almost adult."

"She used to come home and rail against the nuns, remember?" Meg recalled. "Said they were opinionated, bossy and sexually frustrated old women. Guess she was destined to be a contrarian. If we oppose her, you know, she'll get her back up and be even more defiant. But marrying a Jew! That's the limit!"

"How many Jews have you known?" Jack asked, gently.

"Dated one in high school. He was nice enough. He taught me a few things about Jews, mostly about food like bagels and lox, but not really about what he, or they, believed. It didn't go anywhere. My parents were adamant, and it stopped before it even really began."

"I've known several Jews in the building trades. Always had good relations with them. Danny, one of the plumbers I work with, said he had several Jewish friends, knew he could always count on them to come through if he needed them."

Meg was still wrestling with her conflicting emotions. "Maybe we should just meet Ben's parents and see what they think. They might put the kibosh on this marriage anyway and end this whole thing."

"I'll call Mr. Levinson and see if they're willing to talk about this with us," Jack said. "If they are, I'll set a time. Should we meet at their place or ours?"

"Sounds like the right thing to do," Meg said. "Maybe meet them for dinner someplace sorta neutral?"

"I'll call them," Jack said.

~~~

The following Wednesday four nervous adults took their places around a table in a back room at Luca's, an Italian restaurant in the North End. After introductions, Jack asked,

"Does anyone want anything to drink?"

"I'd like some chardonnay," Sophie said. Jacob and Jack shared a bottle of merlot and Meg ordered a gin and tonic. The women ordered the house special, chicken piccata, and the men both got veal scallopini.
~~~

"The most important thing," Sophie said in a lilting voice as they were ordering, "is what we have for dessert!"

"Oh, I dunno," laughed Jack. "I think the main course is the most important."

After the drinks arrived, they looked at one another and sipped their drinks.

"So happy to get acquainted with you," Jack said. Jacob answered, "Likewise." Awkwardness hung over the table like smoke, but after a little lubrication with alcohol, they all relaxed. When food came, they all ate eagerly.

"Now that our tummies are full, maybe we should talk about what we came to discuss," Sophie said in her inimitable straightforward fashion. "Do we think those two should get married?"

"I don't think we have much say in it, to be honest," Jack responded quickly. "They seem to be very much in love."

"The two things we need to talk about are the differing religions and Ben's disability," Jacob said, getting down to the business at hand, as was his habit.

"Can we talk about Ben's paralysis first?" Sophie said. "If I were in your shoes that would worry me a lot."

"Will he ever walk again?" Meg asked, agreeing implicitly with Sophie that this was her big question.

"Not likely," Jacob said. "From what the doctors have told us and from what I've been able to read, his paralysis is permanent."

"He seems to be able to do a lot of things, though," Meg said. "We saw his car and all the gadgets he has to make that work. And his ability to maneuver his wheelchair, braces and crutches is impressive."

"I'm so proud of his progress, his determination, his hopefulness. I don't know that I'd be so optimistic if it were me," Sophie said. "His dedication to medicine is also complete. He'll finish his pediatric training soon and he hopes to go on the faculty at the medical school. He's committed to teaching and improving health care in the inner city."

Jacob looked at Sophie with a combination of surprise and admiration. Surprise because he hadn't realized she'd internalized Ben's motives so completely. His admiration arose from recalling how she'd been so disappointed he'd chosen Suffolk over Boston Pediatric Hospital for his internship and residency and now he discerned her total acceptance of that choice.

"I guess my concern," Meg said, "is that Cathy's taking on a lifetime of caring for, um, I guess I don't know how else to say this, a disabled man. Can her love for him embrace all that will be expected of her?"

"I believe it can," Jacob said in quick response. "And he returns her love in full measure. I see no reason to doubt that. My feeling is that they've already come to grips with his paralysis, and for them, it's no longer an issue."

"I agree with that," Meg said and then hesitated for a moment. "But I have another delicate question, sorry to say," Meg muttered almost in a whisper. "Can they have children?"

"Yes," Jacob said with emphasis. "Ben and I have discussed this in full, without going into details. Unless there are factors we don't know about causing sterility in either one of them, they'll have no difficulty getting pregnant."

Without further discussion of this, they agreed implicitly to move on to the other sticky problem.

"That brings us to religion," Jacob forged on. "First, Sophie and I are Reform Jews, that is, we don't adhere to all Orthodox practices. We do observe many Jewish cultural things: holidays, for example, are important family times for us and we observe them; we do sit Shiva to mourn the passing of a loved one. But we believe universalism is a basic moral underpinning in our daily lives, that is, it emphasizes universal principles of most religions and is inclusive of others."

"Now, Jacob is more liberal than I," Sophie said. "But I agree with most of what he just said. I prefer that my grandchildren are raised as Jews. Our religion and our culture could die out if we keep diluting it. But Jacob doesn't think that would happen. What I want and what Cathy and Benji want may not be the same. I have reluctantly come to the conclusion that I must accept what they decide."

It was Jack and Meg's turn.

"I'm not a good Catholic, I'll say that upfront," Jack began. "I don't often go to mass. I haven't been to confession for a while. But it's hard to forget the childhood grilling. I had a lot of that. I rebelled against it big time in high school. Stopped going to church altogether for a while.

"I have many Jewish friends. I know that's kind of a joke with Jews, 'some of my best friends are Jews.' But it's true with me. Raising grandkids as Jews? I think kids should be exposed to different beliefs, then parents should let them choose whatever fits their needs. They could choose atheism, Buddhism, Judaism, Catholicism, Protestantism, whatever.

"I don't have problems with Cathy marrying Ben. The issue of raising their children in a particular belief system is clearly up to them, I think."

Meg twisted her napkin before she spoke.

"I guess Sophie and I are the ones closer to our original religious beliefs. I go to mass every week and to confession. It's part of my life, has been since I was little. I believe in Jesus, his teachings, and that He is the Son of God." She looked at Jack. "I don't like some things the Church does. It think it's wrong not to allow women to become priests. I think over the centuries the Church has done some awful things. But the Church has done good things too. No religion is perfect. They are all made up of fallible human beings.

"What I'm saying, I guess," Meg continued, "is that Ben and Cathy are deeply in love, and they'll work these things out, just as we all have worked out problems in our relationships. The rest of us will have to deal with our own feelings and help these two however we can."

They left the restaurant together, but each had private reflections about what had just transpired. The four nervous adults who earlier had gotten together to speak of their deepest worries, had listened to each other intently, experienced mutual fears and feelings, and found more common ground than any one of them had expected.

Chapter 33

Drs. Merkel, Crocker, and Zack, 1956

"Adam, got some news for you," Ben said to Adam over lunch at Billy's.

"I think I know what your news is," Adam said with a grin.

"Cathy and I are getting married in July."

"I knew it! That's great news!" he said as he leapt up and came over to Ben's wheelchair, giving him a kiss on his head. "Not a huge surprise, though. When?"

"July 10th."

"Where?"

"Interesting question. We've joined the Norton Street Unitarian Church in Boston. It seemed like a logical choice for a Jew and a Catholic who want to be married and want to avoid the complications of mixed religious services."

"And what do the parents think?"

"They're happy we're getting married. At least that's what they tell us. I'm taking that at face value."

"What about the Unitarian thing?"

"Each of them is a little disgruntled about that for different reasons, but like all compromises, they accepted it as our decision. They've been very decent about it."

Both men sat quietly for a minute. Adam wasn't sure of what to say regarding this weighty turn of events.

"Will you be my best man?" Ben said, breaking the silence.

Tears filled Adam's eyes.

"I'd be honored," he said. "Thank you."

It was Ben's turn to shed a tear.

"Thank you, it's more my honor. Think your girlfriend could come up for the wedding?"

"Well, now that you asked, she's no longer my girlfriend."

"Adam. You didn't tell me. I'm sorry. What happened?"

"You know the old saying, 'Absence makes the heart grow fonder...for somebody else.' It's hard to keep the fire burning when you're apart. It's okay. I'm getting over it. It's been a couple of months now."

"Still a downer though."

"Yep. Let's talk about something else."

"Okay, are you gonna take the faculty position they offered you?" Ben asked.

"Of course. Are you?"

"Definitely. Perfect for me. I'm used to this place, know all the nooks and crannies of the tunnels and floors, how to get around with my chair. Plus, I like everyone here."

"I do too. Dr. Freidman suggested I be the director of the pediatric emergency room. I love the action in the ER. So, I told him to sign me up."

"He wants me to head up the clinics," Ben said. "He's restructuring the whole outpatient department since Dr. Lyons is retiring. So, we'll be working hand in glove!"

~~~

The wedding was well-attended. Both families had large numbers attending and the hospital gang showed up in impressive numbers. After the reception, Ben and Cathy left for a week in Bermuda, courtesy of the four parents. By now, Ben was adept at getting around airports and into airplanes. Stewardesses, once seeing his wheelchair, catered to his every need.

When they got back from their blissful honeymoon, Cathy returned to school, and Ben started his new job.

"How do you like living over the restaurant?" Cathy asked Ben one day.

"Okay for now."

"Hmm. Not an enthusiastic endorsement. Sounds like you maybe would like another place," Cathy said wistfully. "I'd miss this place. We'll never have better neighbors."

"I'd miss it too," Ben said, realizing he now had only one of two votes. "Our own little nest where we
~~~

first made love." His mind wandered back to those halcyon days of early romance, days of lazy sleep-in mornings and the glow of rapturous sex. He then thought of his, what should he call it, his apartment, created by the two other people who loved him best. "I've been spoiled with my pad at home. When my folks remodeled that room for me, they thought of every convenience I could possibly want and need. Don't get me wrong, though, I don't want us to live there. That wouldn't work. I'd like a place we can call our own."

"Well, I'll check the bulletin board at school, where all kinds of things are advertised. Maybe I'll find something there," Cathy said.

"Yeah, I'll do the same at the hospital," Ben said. *Am I being too self-centered? She's lived here for quite a while. I'd better soft-pedal this one a while.*

Back at the hospital, Ben got a call from a nurse on the fourth floor. "Dr. Levinson, there's another case of lead poisoning on our ward. Everyone knows you're interested in this. Can you come up and talk with the residents?"

"I need to finish what I'm doing but I'll be up in about 30 minutes," Ben said "Glad you called. You're right, I am interested in these lead cases."

When he got there, he saw a beautiful three-year-old girl with corn-rolls, large dark eyes, the whites reddened by crying, writhing in pain, and holding her tummy.

"Her X-rays show opacities scattered in her abdomen," a resident said. "Hasn't had a bowel movement in four days, according to mom. She told us she eats peeling paint off the windowsills where they live. When mom sees her doing this, she tries to stop her. But the kid sneaks it when mom's not watching. Blood lead level is 45 micrograms/milliliter. No seizures, but she's very irritable."

"X-rays of her knees?"

"Growth arrest lines. Radiologists called these lead lines. Both sides."

"Have you started EDTA?"

"Yeah, underway. But she's very uncomfortable, and as I said, hasn't had a BM for several days, so we wondered, should we give her a laxative?"

"No, that'll make her cramping worse, but a stool softener might help. Enemas if there are no bowel movements after a couple more days.

"Are there any other kids in this home?" Ben asked.

"They're all older."

"Their lead levels should be checked anyway. Someone gone to the house to find the source?"

"We've contacted the local office of the US Public Health Service. They apparently have equipment that can find lead in houses."

"Thanks for calling me. You're doin' a good job. Keep it up."

As Ben went back to his office, he couldn't get his mind off that little girl, and all the others with this problem. He called Adam.

"Do you think we ought to go to the Department of Public Health? There are these older houses all over the city. We should ask what they can do about it. Whadaya think?"

"Interesting idea. I was talking to Merkel, the head honcho of hematology. Kids with lead poisoning are anemic, as you know. He's been worried about this for some time. I bet we could get him involved in meeting with the Health Department."

"Could you ask him?"

"Sure. You know, maybe we could get a couple of med students interested, stimulate their interest in public health."

"Know any?"

"There are two on the Heme/Onc service now. They look lost most of the time on rounds. I'll talk to them."

"We need a strategy. Maybe Dr. Merkel could meet with us."

A week later they met in the hematology conference room. Dr. Merkel, chief of hematology, had a reputation for being impatient to the point of rudeness, so Ben and Adam were nervous. The two third-year medical students that Adam had recruited, Danny O'Brien and Al Rosen, sat like statues against the wall of Merkel's conference room. Ben and Adam were at the table with Merkel, in his customary long white lab coat. Merkel had grown up in Germantown, Ohio and his attire suggested conservative tastes in dress as well as demeanor. He had a paisley tie tied in a small knot, snugged up in the collar of a blue starched shirt. His dark brown hair was carefully parted in the middle of his head atop his six-foot frame. His nose was slightly off-center, and scuttlebutt had it that it got broken in a college bar fight that he'd started over a snide comment about his German heritage. His greenish eyes were set deep in his face, and when he looked your way, his look seemed to burn into you.

"What's your agenda for this meeting?" he said with pure Teutonic efficiency, wasting no time.

"First we should talk about the rising numbers of lead poisoning cases we're seeing in the hospital," Ben said. "Then we should ask how the Health Department might address this as a public health problem."

"You got statistics about this?" Merkel asked.

"Well, no statistics, just seeing more cases than before," Ben answered.

"Not good enough. We need data, evidence. They won't pay a particle of attention unless we demonstrate with data what our concerns are."

Ben realized that he'd jumped the gun.

"So, get some data," Merkel snapped. "Go to medical records, find out the number of cases in the last couple of years and compare that with this year's numbers. That's a starting point. Then assess the severity of cases. Give them any number, like grades 1,

2 and 3, so we have a rough measure of the severity of cases past and present. Compare the clinical, lab and X-ray findings, especially blood lead levels. You know, there isn't much in the literature about pediatric lead poisoning. This is all publishable if you do it right. Bring the raw data back to me and I'll help you put it together.

"Let's meet again in two weeks. In the meantime, I'll call the commissioner and schedule a meeting in, say a month? Think you can get data together by then?"

Turning to Danny and Al, Ben said, "Can you do this that soon?"

"We're on heme/onc now. Dr. Merkel, can you free us up?" they asked meekly.

"Hell, yes. You can learn a lot by doing this, more than you'll learn tagging along on rounds."

"Okay," Ben said, turning to face Danny and Al. "I'll call the record room and tell them who you are and that you're coming to do this. Can I use your name, Dr. Merkel, to add some prestige to the project?"

"Better still, I'll call the record room and tell them to help you. They know me there. The other thing is, I spoke with Jack Crocker. He's a developmental neurologist and runs a program for brain-related disabilities."

Merkel then fell into his stilted teaching mode. "Lead poisoning in young children has a deleterious effect on their cognitive development, only recently the subject of research." Realizing he was being overly didactic, he got back on track. "Jack is interested in helping you. Call him.

"See you back here in two weeks," Merkel said. The meeting was over. Twelve minutes after it started.

Ben was gratified that the meeting had gone so well and called Dr. Crocker, already alerted to expect his call. He picked right up when he heard it was Ben.

"Thanks for calling, Ben. Glad you're interested in this," Crocker said. "Charles told me of your interest, and I'd like to help. Let's meet and hash out a plan."

"Wonderful. Can I bring a couple of med students and another colleague also interested in this?" Ben asked.

"Sure. Get back to me with a time. I'm game for this."

They met in Crocker's office, once a private home several blocks from County Hospital. It was an old bowfront brick structure, three stories high, with six stone steps leading up to a carved oaken door with original brass fittings. Ben needed Adam and Al to lift him up the stairs and into the vestibule. Off this entry was a conference room, a converted parlor with a large mantle and fireplace on the outside wall. Pocket doors closed off this room from adjoining offices where the clacking typewriters spoke of work going on.

Crocker, a gaunt man with a pipe clenched in his tobacco-stained teeth, came into the room with fragrant cherry tobacco smoke trailing him. Smiling, he removed the pipe from his mouth and greeted them.

"Thanks for coming, and for your interest in lead poisoning and child development. A rare pleasure to see such attention from fellow faculty, and especially from students. Lead poisoning is an invisible toxin. That must change if we're going to protect kids from it. So, let's get started."

Danny and Alan got right to work, exciting for many reasons, not the least of which was because it was outside of the usual scut work assigned to medical students.

In the medical records room, they befriended the librarian and made short work of their assignment. Within four days, they'd gotten data about the last three years of inpatient cases of lead poisoning. They were eager to present their findings to Merkel, Ben, and Adam.

Meeting again in Merkel's office, Alan presented their findings. "Three years ago, the total number of cases for that year was 27, two years ago it was 41, and last year it was up to 62," Dan said. "The youngest cases were in the range of 16 to 20 months, the oldest was 65 months. There was a slight seasonal influence: the peak was in the colder months, when kids were in their apartments more. We graded the severity and there was no significant difference from year to year."

He flipped the page of his report, nervously dropping one page, but recovering it quickly.

"We asked the question: was the rising incidence because of truly increasing incidence or because the diagnosis was being recognized more often? No way to answer that by looking at the data, but it remains a good question." He turned to Dr. Merkel. "Is there an answer to that?"

"It could be that rising awareness made the clinicians test more often for lead poisoning, but that won't be apparent by looking at the raw numbers. We do know anecdotally that in medicine generally that after a Grand Rounds where a particular disease is discussed we see more diagnoses of that disease afterwards. But that doesn't diminish the importance of what you found."

"Thank you, Dr. Merkel," Dan continued, relieved that no criticism or difficult questions came from him. "Several other things were found. There was no worsening of cases in clinical terms, such as levels of blood lead, incidence of serious manifestations such as seizures and anemia. The only thing the data showed was that the numbers were rising each succeeding year."

"Good work, boys," Merkel said, a high compliment from him. Turning to Ben, he said, "I've arranged a meeting with the Commissioner of Public Health for Thursday of next week. Who should be our spokesman?" Merkel asked.

Ben looked at him and Merkel peered back at him intensely. "It's your idea, Dr. Levinson, you should take the lead."

"But I'm a junior faculty member," Ben protested. "Wouldn't either you or Dr. Crocker be a more credible spokesman?"

Merkel considered this for a moment.

"Well, Crocker is most familiar with the long-term effects on cognition, so I can ask him to lead the discussion. Okay?"

Ben quickly agreed.

~~~

Ben went with Crocker and Merkel, who got Ben's wheelchair out of his car. They went into a non-descript Health Department headquarters on Tremont Street in downtown Boston. Inside, the offices were a drab shade of institutional green. He wondered why the Health Department offices were so dismal when their mission was so important. He asked Dr. Merkel about this when he was being ushered into the conference room.

"First, governmental offices all look like this. And the Health Department is low on the totem pole in political importance. The politicians running this city don't give a tinker's damn about the health of the public unless some scandal comes up that could hurt their own reputations and re-election chances," he said. "Unless there's a crisis, they couldn't care less.
~~~

Two years ago, for example, at the height of the polio epidemic, the officials were falling all over themselves to convince the public of their concern. But once that passed, they went on to other things. Government agencies lurch from one emergency to another. This polio epidemic didn't teach them anything to prepare for the next epidemic. It's a real betrayal of trust. Typical."

Ben hoped Merkel's cynicism wasn't reality-based. If he was right, their mission could be doomed from the beginning.

A stale smell from cigarette smoke left over from an earlier meeting met them as they took their seats. A raised platform stood at one end of the room and soon four people filed in and sat in chairs behind a table teetering on the edge of the platform.

"Good morning. I'm Sally Strominger, administrator here at the Department." She introduced two other people and then turned the meeting over to Dr. Zack, Director of Public Health. Sally Strominger was not a large woman, but she towered over Zack, who sat in an elevated chair at the rear of the dais. Ben understood then why they were on the raised dais. Zack needed the elevation to compensate for his small stature. His oversized horn-rimmed glasses dominated the upper half of his face, and his thin lips opened only slightly as he spoke.

"Good morning and welcome. I'm Dr. Elliott Zack. Will you please introduce yourselves?"

Crocker rose and said, "Thank you, Dr. Zack. You probably remember me from previous meetings." Turning to Dr. Merkel, he introduced him as chief of hematology at Suffolk County Hospital. "The man next to him is Dr. Ben Levinson, director of outpatient clinics, and next to him is Dr. Adam Fisher, director of the pediatric emergency room. The two men next to him are medical students from the Charles River University Medical School, Al Rosen and Dan O'Brien."

Crocker then launched into his oft-used lecture about the silent epidemic of lead poisoning. Merkel added his description of lead poisoning-induced anemia. Ben told them about the study Dan and Al did about the rising incidence of lead intoxication over the last three years at County Hospital. When they finished, they looked expectantly at Zack for his response.

"Thank you for caring for children touched by this," Zack said. He glanced at others on the platform. "We talked about this in anticipation of your coming. We don't think lead poisoning is a public health problem in Boston. The cases you're seeing could be seen as instances of parental neglect. However, we appreciate your interest and request you give us a written report of your findings along with data on cognitive developmental delays and anemia. Then we should meet once more after my staff has had time to analyze your data. At the current point in time, however, we are disinclined to mount a public health effort to address this."

Dr. Merkel leaned over to Ben and whispered in his ear, "I've always admired perfection in all its manifestations. Dr. Zack is a perfect jackass."

For his part, Ben was dumbfounded. He leaned over to Merkel to ask his advice about responding. "I'll thank him, and we should leave," he said.

Ben abruptly turned his wheelchair around and headed for the door. The others followed him. In the hall, he was fuming.

"What a miserable little prick!" he cried out.

His intense anger brought back memories of high school, when he often lost his temper at track meets after being pushed out of his running lane. Once he got into a nasty fight with a kid from the other high school. This was the second time Ben had lost his temper and gotten physical with another student. The school was alarmed at his behavior and sent him again for counselling.

He gradually got his anger under better control, but it emerged in situations where he believed someone was being grossly unfair. Zack's response was so dismissive and arbitrary that Ben completely lost his usual calm demeanor and continued to be agitated.

Merkel, surprised by his outburst, reminded of his own anger issues, tried to calm him down.

"Look, we need to develop a more convincing case and come back. Let's talk some more to Crocker and see what he thinks we need to do next, come back, and then if Zack won't respond with a plan of action, we'll get the community involved, go to the newspapers and sound the alarm. I'm now really in this fight."

Chapter 34

Rev. Gordon Hightower

"Frustrating in the extreme," Ben, still sizzling, said to Crocker at their next meeting. "That little jerk really got me goin'."

"Didn't surprise me. Zack has been unhelpful in my previous efforts to shine a light on this problem," Crocker said. "Not the first time I've told him about lead poisoning, only to be ignored. I suspect -- don't quote me outside this room -- he's been warned to keep his hands off. Powerful and well-bankrolled people don't want this can of worms opened. Slum landlords know getting rid of lead paint in their rental units would cost them a bundle. They don't give a damn about poor kids, especially in minority communities."

"So, what should we do next?" Ben asked in a low voice, reflecting his angry mood.

"Document the problem with a wider scope of data," Crocker said. "Meet with community leaders who have credibility with people living there. Go to health centers and collect blood from young kids, test it for lead. Nobody should have lead in their blood.

Publish your data. If that doesn't wake Zack and his Health Department up, go public with it, spread the news."

Ben listened with growing excitement. This was a data-driven medical mission with a social impact. True preventive medicine. Getting rid of the cause of a disease, like killing organisms with antibiotics. Like the vaccine Salk had developed for polio.

"You know any community organizers for County Hospital neighborhoods?" Ben asked.

"I know a man who has a strong influence within the Negro community," Jack said. "Name is Gordon Hightower, a colored minister, a force of nature. His enthusiasm for helping his people is boundless. He's also well known outside of his church. He even has a call-in show on a local radio station. I'll call him. He knows everyone. Maybe he can give you a forum for this message. One other thing. I'll give you the name of a lab where they test blood from industry workers exposed to lead in their jobs. Only problem is that they need 10 milliliters of blood. That's a lot of blood to get out of little people."

"We're used to getting blood from tiny veins," Ben laughed. His mind sparked from one thought to another about what else needed to be done. "A bunch of other things occur to me. One is, can we test their houses while we're at it?"

"That's a little trickier," Crocker said. "But I know a fellow from the US Public Health Service office in town who inspects homes for all kinds of hazardous materials. I'll call him and see if he can help us," Crocker said. "A great companion study."

Ben could hardly wait to get in touch with the Reverend Mr. Gordon Hightower. Adam, however, was a little wary about this idea when Ben told him about Reverend Mr. Hightower.

"My experience with community organizers, admittedly small, is they're full-bore politicians, with more interest in promoting themselves than they have in people in their communities.," he said. "But I'd like to be in on your meetings with him," Adam said. "You say he's a minister? And colored? Interesting. Maybe I'll find some common ground with him."

"I'd like to have you in all our meetings about this," Ben said. "You'll make this effort credible to colored communities."

"Just so you don't go and make me a 'token Negro,'" he said with a serious tone.

Ben wasn't sure what to say. He hesitated, thought about his response, and finally said, "I'll take my cues from you, Adam. You tell me if you think I'm doing the wrong thing."

"Sorry, Ben," picking up on his uncertainty. "I don't mean to throw a wet blanket on this. But I'm real sensitive about racial issues, especially when they're health related. Think of Tuskegee, of Henrietta Lacks. I know about Lacks since I'm from Baltimore. That's where she was mistreated. Don't misunderstand. I believe this is the right thing to do," Adam said, "but I wanna be careful not to presume anything about our research subjects, or the community."

Ben got Reverend Mr. Gordon Hightower's phone number from Jack Crocker and called him. After a few calls, he reached him.

"Reverend Hightower, this is Ben Levinson. I'm a pediatrician at Suffolk County Hospital, very concerned about lead poisoning in children we're seeing here. Dr. Jack Crocker gave me your name as someone who might help us as we try to get a handle on how to approach this."

"What can I do for you?" he said with wariness.

Ben told him about the rising numbers of kids seen in the hospital with lead poisoning and his idea to test the blood for lead on vulnerable child populations in communities adjacent to Suffolk Hospital.

"I need someone who's known and trusted in the community to explain why this problem is so important to them as parents. We need their trust to give permission for us to collect blood from their kids to test it for lead. We hope you'd be willing to help us."

A long silence at the other end of the line made Ben nervous, but he let the time slide by without saying more.

"I need to talk with you further before I commit," Hightower said. "Can you come and talk to me?"

"Give me some times," Ben said. He couldn't get a sense of Hightower from their brief phone exchange.

Reverend Hightower told him where his church was and gave him several dates. Ben wondered if he should tell him of his disability but decided he would take a cab with Adam who could accompany him and help him navigate. He called him and they agreed on a time.

Ben and Adam found Hightower's church on Warren Street. It was a modest but well-maintained wooden structure, painted white, with traditional New England steeple, and an entryway up several steps. Ben snapped on his knee braces, stood up on his crutches, and Adam, with the cab driver's help, got him up the stairs to the front door, leaving his chair at the curb. After knocking on the locked door and getting no answer, Adam went around to the side of the church where he found an unlocked door. He entered and found Reverend Hightower's office. He knocked and Reverend Hightower opened the door. Adam confronted a man as big as he was, but thirty years older, with a linebacker's frame. His face was kindly, a contrast to his threatening size. Their brown eyes met on a level plane.

"Can I help you?" Reverend Hightower said in his almost stereotypically deep sonorous minister's voice. He was momentarily confused, as he faced this other enormous colored guy standing in his doorway.

"I'm Dr. Adam Fisher, Reverend Hightower. Dr. Levinson and I are here to talk to you about our proposed lead poisoning project. I left Ben at the front door of the church. The door is locked." He didn't mention that Ben was unable to walk.

"Oh, I'm sorry. That door stays locked except when we have services. Have a problem with theft around here. Tell him to come around here."

"Could you let him in the front door? You see, he's unable to walk, he uses a wheelchair."

"Oh, for heaven's sake, I didn't know. Sure, I'll open that door and let him in. I'll meet you out there."

When they were all finally in Reverend Hightower's office, he apologized, saying, "If I'd had any idea this would be a problem, I would've met you out front. Sorry."

"I should have told you, but sometimes it's hard for me to talk about my disability. I worry about being pitied," Ben said. "Anyhow, thanks for meeting with us. We're glad to be here. You've already met Adam, my pediatric colleague who runs the pediatric emergency room at the hospital.

"What can I tell you about lead poisoning in children?" Ben asked. "How much do you know?"

"Not much. I've heard talk about kids getting sick from eating paint chips, but I don't know any details. I'd like to hear more if you say it's a problem we have here."

Ben launched straight into describing the problem, the urgent need for screening kids for lead in their blood to prevent the toxin from damaging their developing brains. "We can do the blood testing easily in community health centers. When we find elevated levels, we can treat the kids at the hospital."

Reverend Hightower listened intently to Ben, looking back and forth from him to Adam. When Ben had finished, he sighed, and said, "I've heard bits and pieces about a few kids going into the hospital with stomach aches and being told it was because they were eating peeling paint, but I had no idea it was dangerous to their brains. After you do the blood tests, and whatever else you plan on doing, what then?"

"Our first goal, for obvious reasons, is to treat kids who have any lead in their blood. There is a drug we call EDTA, a so-called chelating agent that binds the lead so it can be safely excreted by the kidneys without damaging their brains. We do that in the hospital. But, you know, those kids shouldn't go back to houses where they got it in the first place. Lead paint chips taste sweet, and we worry about the kids becoming habituated to the sweet taste. So, the next step is to go to those houses, find the lead, and make it unavailable to the kids."

"How?"

"That's the big question. Paint can be sanded off, you know, but permissions to do that has to come from landlords, who won't allow it unless they're forced to. Sanding costs lots of money, must be done by highly trained personnel, taking all kinds of precautions to prevent the dust from being inhaled by anyone in the vicinity of the sanding. The workers who do this wear special protective clothing and masks themselves and have periodic blood tests to check their blood for lead. During sanding, families must live somewhere else. Inhalation of airborne paint dust is even more dangerous than eating paint chips."

"Sounds to me like laws are needed to make lead paint illegal. And housing laws forcing landlords to make the units safe. You're tackling a big, complicated problem."

"You're right. Making lead paint illegal is important, for sure, but the fact is that practically all houses and apartments built before World War-II have lead paint in them. It was always considered the best paint. Making lead-based paint illegal makes sense, and we should pursue that, but it doesn't solve the present problem -- where the paint already is."

"You've certainly got my interest," Reverend Hightower said. He gazed up at the ceiling, in deep thought, and then said, "I think I can help. I can publicize this project on my radio show and urge mothers to bring their little ones to their health centers for lead testing and get treated if the levels are up." Reverend Hightower was a quick study. "I also have a large congregation -- the biggest in the community -- and I can use my bully pulpit to get the word out. After that, what do you want me to do?"

"After we have data, we need to go back to the Health Department and ask them for help to address this. It is, after all, a public health problem. Perhaps you could join us at that meeting and help us advocate for a public health effort to stop this silent epidemic. If they don't help, we'll need to figure out what other avenues we can pursue. And you could help there, using your radio show."

Ben looked at Adam. "Did I miss anything?"

"Yeah, a couple of things. We have two medical students who want to help. They'll go to health centers themselves to personally draw the blood. They have lots of experience doing this in the hospital, so mothers can be assured they're experienced and good at this. The other thing is, with students doing the blood tests, health center personnel won't feel they're being overwhelmed with new tasks.

"The important thing for everyone to know is that we'll explain to mothers the way lead hurts their kids," Adam said. "They can choose not to participate if they don't think this will help their kids. And we'll give the results of testing to them just as soon as we know them. They need to feel they're included in the process. Most importantly, we don't want moms thinking their kids are being used as guinea pigs"

"Well, this is very informative," Reverend Hightower said. "Thanks. What's the next step?"

"Getting the word out in the community to get their kids tested and how to access this service," Ben said. "Dr. Crocker, our mental disabilities expert, has some money in his budget for this kind of project, so this will be free to the mothers.

"Your endorsement would help a lot, Reverend Hightower. If you talk about this on your show, get people's interest and cooperation, we'll do the rest. We'll need to get the health centers on board. They'll recognize the need for this, I believe. If they don't, we'll work on convincing them. But I don't see that as an obstacle.

"We'll get written materials ready for you to read on your show, hand out or post wherever they'll be seen -- in grocery stores, in health center waiting rooms, other churches, take-out restaurants, and the like. We'll set up a schedule for testing when we get further along."

"Sounds good. But you should come on my show and talk about this project. I'm interested in helping. Let me know when I can count on you for the show," Hightower said.

As they left, Adam turned to Ben.

"I'm impressed with Reverend Hightower. Sorry I was skeptical. He's a good man. I trust him. This is getting exciting. Can't wait to get it going.

"I have something else to tell you," Adam said in a conspiratorial tone.

"Uh-oh. What?"

"I've been seeing too many cases of what I think are child abuse in the ER. I've been thinking about this awful problem and researching what little is written about how different hospitals are responding to it. I have an idea, based on some models I've read about."

"Sounds interesting. Tell me more."

"Some hospitals, mainly children's hospitals, are forming what they call 'multidisciplinary teams' or MDT's. The teams consist of a doctor, a nurse, and a social worker, sometimes others. The MDTs are on call to consult with the docs in the ER or inpatient services who're suspicious the injuries they're seeing could be non-accidental, that is, inflicted, or if there's child neglect. They work with providers to decide what to do -- appropriate tests to perform, such as X-rays or blood tests for toxic substances, screening for other health issues like anemia, malnutrition, general hygienic deprivation -- that sort of thing. What do you think?"

"Great idea, another thing that falls under the rubric of social pediatrics, the play of social conditions on health. How can I help?"

"Well, I guess your outpatient department could also use these consultations. And if you want to be on the team, we'd love that too."

"I'm game. Count me in. We should also incorporate this topic in our lecture series to residents and medical students. Is there a literature on this?"

"Not much, and that's the other thing I want to do. Conduct studies to define this phenomenon and get something into the pediatric literature to educate others how to deal with it. We might get non-profit foundation grants to underwrite studies."

"Are there any books on this?" Ben asked, his curiosity aroused.

"Not yet, and that's another one of my goals. To publish a textbook for diagnosing and treating child abuse and neglect."

Ben again admired these qualities in his friend. He was always finding new ways to help his patients.

"Adam, I'm one of your greatest fans. I'm with you, 100 percent!"

Chapter 35

House Hunting, Cathy's News

"I just was called by a realtor," Ben said to Cathy. "She has a property near the hospital that she says is a 'steal,' as she put it. "It's one of those beautiful three-story brick buildings that have gone to ruin over the years. The owners are desperate to sell. It needs lots of work, but it has, as she puts it, 'good bones.' You interested in seeing it?"

"How did she know to call you?" were the first words out of Cathy's mouth.

Chagrined that he'd been found out doing some sleuthing about a property they could buy, he said, "Well, I've talked with her before and told her we might be in the market for a property if one cropped up. I didn't mention it because I didn't think she'd find something so quickly. You mad at me? I can call her and tell her we're not interested."

"No, I'm not mad at you," Cathy chuckled. "Just surprised. I know you want our own place. I guess I do too. I'm just so attached to my little place." After considering the possibility of a new place to live, she said, "I guess there's no harm in looking."

They met Jane Cotton, the realtor, late Friday afternoon just before Thanksgiving. It was just cool enough that they could see their breath and needed light jackets. Cathy looked at the property from the street and could see possibilities. It was a handsome old building with bay windows in the bow-front on all three stories. There were six stone steps up to the landing in front of an old mahogany door needing some serious help. Ben couldn't get up those steps to go inside, but Cathy accompanied Jane inside. Cathy, the daughter of an electrician, had some experience with the world of rehabilitation of old housing stock.

What she saw was a living space inside on three floors with heavy bannisters and balustrades providing access to each floor, all needing refinishing. The living room, dining room and kitchen on the first floor were large rooms with original oak floors needing sanding and new varnish. The kitchen at the rear of the house was in serious disrepair. Three upstairs bedrooms were spacious, and the front windows gave plenty of light to the front room, but the back two bedrooms had exterior windows only on one side, this unit being the corner unit of the block. The bathroom was a disaster. The third floor was unfinished but could be made into two more bedrooms.

"The asking price is only $30,000. Taxes are low because it's where it is, here in the South End," Jane said. "That's why I told you this was a steal. You can see it's gonna take a lot of rehab to make it livable, but it's a potentially a great property."

"I see its potential," Ben said. "But I can also see big problems for me. Getting in and out of that building would be a daily challenge for me. And getting from floor to floor. I like the location. For me it's ideal, it's so close to the hospital. For you, Cathy, it would require commuting to the Channing School." Turning to Jane, Cathy said, "How about parking?"

"One dedicated spot on the street. As you can see, this street is divided by a ten-foot, tree-lined lawn, the whole distance to the next cross street. That's shared and deeded property. Everyone on the street owns it. There's an alley behind all the buildings and rear entrances. I can visualize an elevator on the outside of the building, on the alley side, to get you to all the floors inside. You'd never have to use the front entry."

"What about schools?" Cathy asked, surprising Ben.

"Well, you'd probably want to consider private schools. I didn't know you had kids," Jane said.

"We don't, yet," Cathy said.

"We'll talk it over and get back to you," Ben told Jane. "It would be a stretch, and we'd have to know a lot more about this place. Cathy's father is an electrician and could look at it if we're interested. I'll call you."

As soon as they were alone, Ben said, "Why did you ask about schools?"

"I was going to tell you this week," Cathy said, with a mischievous grin. "I'm pregnant."

Ben's face flushed, he smiled broadly, reached up and pulled Cathy onto his lap in his wheelchair, kissed and hugged her, both laughing uncontrollably.

"When did you find out?" Ben said, when he was finally calm enough to talk.

"Last Friday. I went to Dr. Lane, and he confirmed it."

"When are you due?"

"In June. Early June."

"Can we tell the parents?" Ben asked.

"Let's wait until we're sure the pregnancy is a little further along. Miscarriages happen," Cathy said in her pragmatic way.

They went home to Cathy's apartment and had dinner in the Ethiopian restaurant downstairs.

"Hi, how are you, so glad to see you," the waiter said with a wide smile as they came in. "Sit in usual place?"

Once seated, Ben studied the menu, then looked up at Cathy. "I'm so happy, I can hardly focus on food. Tell him I want the usual. I can't even remember what that is."

Laughing, she ordered the same, and they looked at each other in the soft light. Both got misty.

"It changes things, you know," Ben said.

"Well, sure it does, but what exactly do you mean?"

"We can't buy that place in the South End. Not with a baby coming. That's a major project and is not really the kind of place we need. I liked it, and it's really neat, but looking at it with a cold eye, it's not really for us, I don't think. What do you think?"

"I'm so glad you feel that way. I looked at that building and saw work, work, and more work to make it livable. Can you imagine how expensive the rehab would be on that place? And we'd definitely need that elevator for you."

"And with a new baby? My God, no way. Just getting in and out of the place would be a challenge, not only for me but for you too. With baby carriages, with groceries, laundry -- we didn't even think of that, and God knows how many other things." Ben looked at Cathy and considered still other concerns that old building provoked in him.

"You remember my lead poisoning project? That building is probably loaded with lead, in addition to all the other stuff we're now thinking about. I think we need to keep looking. We can stay here at your apartment until a couple of months before you deliver, okay? By the way, did Dr. Lane refer you to an OB?"

"He told me he doesn't do deliveries anymore, so yes, he referred me to an obstetrician he knows at the Lying-In Hospital."

"I'm glad. It's better to have an OB anyway. I like Dr. Lane, I've known him since I was little, but if something went wrong, I'd want the best doctor there is to take care of you."

The food came and their excitement had made them extra hungry. They ate voraciously with no conversation until the plates were empty, then they gazed at each other with fresh eyes, both realizing their lives had changed still again. New responsibilities. Wonderment about new life. Finding a new home. Lots to think about.

Chapter 36

Revisiting the Health Department

December 1956–January 1957

"Adam, Reverend Hightower asked us to be on his radio show. Exactly what we need to kick this off," Ben said, his voice in high spirits. "I've lined up four community health centers, two in Roxbury and two in Dorchester, to use their facilities. We can go on his show to publicize what I've dubbed 'roundup days' at the health centers."

"That's terrific! When's our debut?" Adam asked, mirroring Ben's excitement. Ben told him the date and they chose the dates for the "round-up."

Hightower's show usually opened with his monologue, followed by a guest speaker and a call-in segment. Today, he began with a description of an anonymous case of lead poisoning to introduce his guests.

"Adeline is a delightful five-year-old girl who loves to play hopscotch and is looking forward to starting first grade in September. She already reads a lot of kid books even though she never has been to school. Her mom has taught her that.

"But Adeline has a problem her mom can't seem to control. She loves to eat peeling paint chips in their apartment. Why? Her mom found out the paint chips are sweet. She asked her pediatrician at the hospital about this habit. He told her the paint chips taste sweet because they have lead acetate in them. Lead acetate is in most paints used in houses before the war. The really bad part of this is that when lead goes to the child's developing brain it can cause irreversible damage."

He glanced at Ben and Adam and nodded.

"Today's guests are two doctors from Suffolk County Hospital to talk about a program they're working on to detect lead poisoning and to prevent the brain damage it causes. Dr. Ben Levinson and Dr. Adam Fisher, welcome to my program. I'm eager to learn more about this threat to our little children."

"Thanks, Reverend Hightower, we appreciate the opportunity to discuss this with your listeners," Ben said.

He then outlined what he wanted to do and asked the listening audience to help them test their kids for lead poisoning. Adam followed by identifying the four locations at health centers they'd lined up to be testing centers.

After the show and thanking Reverend Hightower, Adam said, "I'd like to test around 250 kids between one and six years old. Then we'll have hard data for the Health Department. And after we analyze the data and figure out what we have, we can publish our results."

"That's a lot of kids! Any idea how many will have elevated lead?" Reverend Hightower asked.

"I'm not gonna stick my neck out on that. What do you think, Ben?"

"Me neither. Interesting to get real figures. We should test the houses too."

"Good thought, geez, I forgot about that. I'll call the Public Health Service guy, you know, whose name Dr. Crocker gave me, who tests homes for lead. We also need a statistician to help us, and I'll ask my secretary to try to keep track of all this stuff," Ben was reeling these things off as he thought of them. "I've never done research before, so we'll have to feel our way along. We need all the help we can get to do it right."

Their plan was crystallizing. They set the testing days for January. Reverend Hightower, an amazingly resourceful man, found a taxi company in Mattapan who offered free transportation for mothers who had no way to get to the health centers.

By the end of January, they had collected bloods on 240 children. Roger Bailey, Crocker's contact from the Public Health Service, had gotten into the homes of those kids whose lead levels were up. The project had gone more smoothly than anyone could have imagined. They compiled their results and submitted their paper to Childhood Diseases, a leading pediatric journal.

Drs. Merkel and Crocker were ecstatic about the success of this endeavor. So were Ben, Adam and the medical students who drew all the blood samples. Nearly one quarter of the children tested had high blood lead levels, much higher than expected. In every home of children with elevated lead levels, lead paint was detected using a portable radioisotope X-ray fluorescence analyzer.

"Okay, now we have data. Irrefutable data. If the Health Department won't listen to this, we'll go to the newspapers," Merkel said. "I'll set up another meeting with them."

"Can't wait to see my old friend Dr. Zack," Ben chuckled. "We need the Health Department to understand that we have a lead poisoning problem in this city.

"We need to treat the kids with high lead, of course," Ben said to Merkel. "I got permission from our chairman to create a toxicology clinic for that. There, in addition to treatment, we can teach mothers some ways to keep their kids from further ingestion. Unfortunately, we can't just move them from their houses, so we have to make lead paint chips unavailable to them," Ben was on a roll. "Paint over the old paint? Put masking tape over it? I don't know the answers to those questions yet." He couldn't stop talking, he was so excited. Merkel smiled in satisfaction as he listened.

"We're also considering setting up a local Poison Information Center for parents to call when their kids have ingested medicines, or bleach, or mineral spirits, and many other things that can harm them. I've called several hospitals in the state, and no one has a poison center. So, this is the starting point for a lot of neat new programs."

~~~

They went to the Health Department in early February, to the same dingy room they were in before. This time, however, no Dr. Zack. In his place was a Dr. Mary Agnew, the deputy Health Commissioner. No reason was given for his absence. *That bastard doesn't even show up for this follow-up meeting. Shows his lack of interest in our effort.*

Sally Strominger introduced Dr. Agnew. She was a diminutive middle-aged woman with brown short-cropped hair and a soft, low-pitched speaking voice. Dr. Crocker began by thanking them for holding the meeting, then turned the meeting over to Ben and Adam.

"Since our last meeting, much has been accomplished. We'd like to present the results of our project." Ben laid out the materials and methods of their study, gave the results highlighting that nearly 25% of the 240 kids between one and six years of age
~~~

from the neighborhoods around Suffolk County Hospital had high blood lead levels, and that all the homes in which these children lived were tested and found to have lead paint on windowsills and other woodwork. "We concluded that, at least in these neighborhoods, there is a major public health problem of lead poisoning affecting children between one and six years old." He paused for effect. "We respectfully ask you, the Health Department, to respond to this silent epidemic with an action plan."

There was dead silence in the room as Ben finished. This, combined with Zack's absence, didn't bode well. He turned to Adam and asked if he had further comments.

"Yes. We did this study because we saw rising numbers of lead poisoning cases at our hospital over the last three years. We came here a few months ago and were told by Dr. Zack that the Health Department didn't believe there was a lead poisoning problem in our city, and he asked us to provide better information. We've done that. You just heard the results of our study. I think we have a problem. We hope you do too."

Dr. Agnew looked at Ben and Adam. "Very impressive piece of work you've done. I believe your results prove we do have a public health problem in addition to a medical one. Thank you for doing this."

Well, now, this sounds better. Wonder where Zack is and whether he'd agree with this, Ben thought.

"Addressing this comprehensively is our job. It won't be easy and won't happen overnight, but I'll advocate for putting this on an urgent basis. As you might anticipate this will require money. That must come from the county and perhaps also the state legislature. As Acting Health Commissioner, I'll be in touch with the County Commissioners today to put this on a fast track to provide funds for testing and treatment of pediatric lead poisoning."

Ben looked at Adam, then Dr. Merkel and Dr. Crocker when he heard "Acting Health Commissioner." Did this mean Eliot Zack was no longer the Commissioner? They all suppressed their glee at this news, keeping poker faces but laughing inside. Ben could hardly wait to get outside to let out a whoop.

"I'll get back to you after I've talked with the county folks, and we've developed a plan of action. Thank you once more for your efforts. I hope we will have good news for you in the near future."

After this meeting, Ben thrust his arm into the air, whirled his chair around in a circle, and cried "All right! We were heard!" The temptation of the group was to go immediately to the Bean and Cod Bistro to celebrate, but they had to get back to work. They shook hands and agreed a victory party could wait until they heard from Dr. Agnew after her meeting with the appropriate county and state officials.

Chapter 37

A Better Bet, March 1957

"Guess what?" Cathy said when Ben called. He could barely wait to tell her about their meeting, but she pre-empted the conversation. He was apprehensive when she opened the conversation that way but waited to hear what she had to say.

"I've possibly found a house for us," she said with a lilt in her voice. "In West Roxbury, one-floor plan, with garage and beautiful back yard and deck. Three bedrooms, one-and-half baths, and, shall we say, an 'adequate' kitchen."

"Really? How'd you find it?" Ben's heart rate sped up, suppressing his excitement about telling her about their meeting.

"On the bulletin board here at Channing. I called right away. We can see it this weekend. What do you think of that?"

"That's great! You say we can see it this weekend?"

"Yeah, and the other thing, it's within walking distance to an elementary school!"

"I'll be damned. Good work, my dear wife," Ben said. "So glad we didn't fall in love with that house in the South End. It was a great building, but not for us.

"I've got some good news too," Ben said, bursting with eagerness to tell her about the meeting.

"Is it about the Health Department?"

"Yep. They actually listened. They have a new Acting Commissioner who looks like she's gonna advocate for this program for the city. She'll be talking to the powers that be today. We hope this'll mean support for our project. Money support as well as philosophical support."

"Oh, that's wonderful, Ben. So happy for you. I know how hard you've worked on this. Can't wait to see you. So, we have two things to be excited about."

"When can we look at this place?" Ben's long suit had never been patience.

"I'll call her and see if we can see it Saturday." Ten minutes later Cathy called back. The appointment was for set for Saturday at ten.

They were both excited, waking early on Saturday in the apartment. Ben drove the Suburban, wondering if the garage at this house would be big enough for this gigantic car. He also worried about access into the house. Cathy told him it was on one floor, so he wasn't concerned about navigating inside. But getting into any house was always a problem. In Chestnut Hill, Jacob and Sophie had designed his room for easy access and plenty of handrails and lift devices. He'd been so spoiled, and he knew it. He prayed the entry to this house would be on level ground.

They arrived before Jocelyn, the real estate agent, so Ben left the motor running to keep warm. He scanned the house from the street. Uh-oh. There were five stairs to the porch in the front entrance. "Where's the garage?" he asked Cathy. "Can you see it?"

"I don't see it. It must be in the back. Worried about those stairs?" Cathy asked, knowing the answer.

"Yeah, doesn't look good. This house hunting may take time. Whoever designs houses hasn't counted on people like me," he groused. "Another cause for me to address."

"Ben, you can't change everything wrong with the world single-handedly," Cathy chided him. "Besides, you haven't seen the whole house. One thing, before we go inside, I want to warn you that Jocelyn told me the kitchen needed some help. But that can be fixed. The entry problem is another matter."

Jocelyn rolled up and parked behind them. She jumped out of the car and waved to them, indicating they should meet her on the front porch. Cathy waved back and hurried to catch up to her. Ben watched as they had an animated conversation. She came back to the car.

"Drive into the driveway and around to the back of the building. Stop in front of the garage door. Jocelyn and I will meet you there."

He did as he was told and headed towards the garage door, which opened just as he approached it. Jocelyn waved to him to drive into the garage. The Suburban fit with a couple of inches overhead to spare. The garage was big enough for two cars. Ben breathed a sigh of relief.

"Hi, I'm Jocelyn," she said with enthusiasm, in true realtor fashion. "You can get out here. The door into the house is right over there," she said pointing to a door leading, as Ben found out, into the kitchen. Ben emerged from the car, snapped on his knee braces, got his crutches, and followed Jocelyn and Cathy into the house. Cathy ran back to get his wheelchair out of the Suburban. As he watched her get his chair out, he thought about her pregnancy and decided that in a few months he shouldn't let her lift that heavy chair.

"I should have told you to drive around back, but I didn't expect you so early," Jocelyn said. "I'm sorry about those steps to the front porch. No one told me about your walking problem." She didn't say that with blame in her voice, only regret that she didn't know. Ben smiled, feeling reassured he could get into the house from the garage with no problem.

It was, as Cathy had warned, a dismal kitchen, with the 1940's jumping out everywhere they looked. The refrigerator and stove were an ugly green, the cabinets orange, the linoleum floors were worn thin, and the sink stained with rust and gray residue. But the room was large, had twin windows over the sink looking out to a pleasant backyard with a big lawn surrounded by mature rhododendrons.

As they moved from one room to another, Cathy seemed to warm to this house. Ben was unsure this was "it" as he gazed around, trying to visualize what it would be like living here, but he was aware that he had zero experience in house-shopping. None. Once they were finished looking and back in their van, Ben said, "Well, what do you think?"

"There were some good things about it, and some not so good. I'd like Dad to see it and tell me what he thinks. He knows houses better than anyone I know."

"Good idea. Let's call him and see when he could take a look. Is there any hurry? Will someone else snap this place up if we piddle around?"

"Sooner the better. I'll call him when we get home."

Jack was glad she'd called. He loved looking at houses and was good at assessing their worth. "I have time tomorrow," Jack said, glad to be able to help in this big decision. "Call the realtor and set a time."

They agreed on a time: Sunday at one. Jack asked if Meg could come along.

"Of course. She'll have ideas about the kitchen," Cathy said, looking at Ben. "Do you think your folks should come too?"

"Oh, yes, definitely, we should ask them. If we don't, they'd be very peeved. If they can't come tomorrow, we can arrange another time. I'll call them."

The next day at the house Jocelyn was surprised and somewhat daunted by the family but hopeful this augured well for a sale. Jack did his inspection, Sophie and Meg consulted about the kitchen and Jocelyn watched, hoping they'd make an offer. She thought the price was right and she liked this couple and their parents.

"Can you all come to our house for dinner and talk? We can have take-out Chinese," Sophie said to Jack and Meg before they left.

Ben called the restaurant, and they gathered at Jacob and Sophie's. Ben glanced at his room wistfully when they got there. It was such a godsend when he was battling the first stages of his recovery.

"What does everyone think?" Cathy asked as soon as they began eating. "I can't wait to hear!"

"Well, Meg and I have already redesigned the kitchen," Sophie laughed. "We don't think it will take a whole lot."

"I respectfully disagree," Jack said with a smile. "It'll cost a lot. But it's doable. The rest of the house seems fine, no big problems. I saw a couple of small things that need fixing. The electrical system needs upgrading, not unusual in houses this age. But overall, not a bad house."

"How old is it?" Jacob asked.

"Built in '35, according to Jocelyn," Cathy said.

"Did anyone see anything seriously wrong with it?" Ben asked. No one spoke up.

"Are we rushing things?" Ben said.

"Was the asking price right?" Jacob asked, ever the businessman.

"About right, I think." Jack said. "I don't know the market in West Rox, but the price seems in line with places I work in."

Turning to Ben and Cathy, Jacob said, "Can you swing this?"

They looked at each other. "I don't know," Cathy said, her hand on her forehead. "We'll have to look at our finances."

"It's not as though we both have high-paying jobs, but we both are employed," Ben said. "It'll all depend on our bank. The fact is we must have a place for what will be three of us in June."

"I'm willing to help," Jacob said.

"We are too," Jack chimed in. "And I can find some reasonable craftsmen to do the kitchen."

The conversation lagged as each person was lost in individual contemplation of the various considerations involved. Ben looked at Cathy, who returned his stare. Jack, Meg, Sophie, and Jacob were all looking at their hands or fiddling with what was left of their food, taking a drink, wondering what would be said next, and by whom.

Ben finally broke the silence. "Why don't we all sleep on it and consult tomorrow evening, when we're all home from the real world of work?"

"Good!"

"Fine!"

"I agree!"

"What a day," Ben said as he and Cathy drove home.

"A good day, I say," Cathy replied. "I've already decided what we should do."

"You gonna tell me?"

"We agreed we'd talk tomorrow night. I'm gonna wait until then."

"Well, damn!" Ben chuckled.

Chapter 38

Meeting with Ann McDonough, Legal Department

They regarded each other in the morning cautiously. Ben knew Cathy wasn't going to tip her hand. He thought he knew what it was: Buy! But he knew she was seriously unpredictable, so until she actually said it, he couldn't be sure. He'd just have to wait, not easy for him.

When Ben got to work his secretary told him he had a message from Dr. Friedman to call him as soon as he got in.

"Dr. Friedman, this is Ben Levinson. You called?"

"Yes, come to my office. I need to discuss an important matter with you."

What the hell? That could be good or bad, but what was it?

When he got to Friedman's office his secretary ushered him into his inner sanctum. He was on the phone. He fixed him with his eyes and continued his conversation with -- whom? This was not, however, unusual with Friedman. Ben thought he enjoyed the mystery he created when he conversed by phone with an unknown person while you were in his presence without revealing who and what the discussion was about. When he ended the call, he looked, without any expression at Ben.

"I got a call late yesterday from a lawyer about your lead poisoning project," he began. "He listened to Hightower's radio program and heard what you've done. He represents a group of property owners who are worried this project will cause them a lot of bad press and unhappy tenants. He also said he's in touch with paint manufacturers who've gotten wind of this. They're very upset because they consider the use of lead acetate essential to maintain the high quality of their paint." He looked directly at Ben. "I thought you should know this."

"So, this lawyer actually heard Hightower's program?" Ben asked. "How did he know about it?"

"There are leaks all over the place when threats to business practices arise," he said. "Specifically, there was a shakeup at the Health Department and the former Commissioner is complaining he's the victim of a 'plot' to expose the city's lack of attention to lead poisoning. Sound familiar?"

Ben's stomach was tightening as he realized the imbroglio he'd stirred up. "But we proved that lead poisoning is real. That's a truth that can't be negated. Just because that little jerk is whining that he lost his job because of this, doesn't mean we're wrong."

"Calm down, Ben. I'm not saying you're wrong. I simply wanted you to know this is going on. There are powerful men in this city who don't want their ability to make money compromised. They're not going to take this lying down."

"So, what will your position be?" Ben asked warily.

"I'm standing behind you, of course. I strongly believe in this project. So do Crocker and Merkel. We're all with you on this. So don't worry about that. But we need legal advice. I've set up a meeting with the hospital legal department, so we have guidance for our response. Okay?"

"I appreciate your support and the others as well. When is the meeting?" Ben's voice shook as he spoke. "Who will be at the meeting?"

"I've asked Merkel, Crocker, Adam Fisher, and you to attend. They've all said they can come."

"When?"

"Today at 2:00. In the legal office. Cancel anything else you have this afternoon. See you there."

Ann McDonough was Suffolk's lead attorney and chaired the meeting. After welcoming Ben, Adam, Merkel, and Crocker, she wasted no time.

"First let me say I'm proud to represent our hospital and the doctors addressing this important issue. The lawyer representing the property owners is Michael LaMonte. He's well-known for taking on issues challenging owners' interests. This is a juicy one for him and may lead to others involving the paint manufacturers. So, as usual, money is driving the interests of both."

Ben listened intently but was reluctant to ask questions. Not so, Dr. Merkel.

"They can send up all the fireworks they want, but, as a non-lawyer, I see no basis for a suit. We have simply demonstrated a scientific truth. There are children with lead poisoning, and they live in houses where we've demonstrated the presence of lead."

"You're technically correct, Doctor. They have no grounds for a suit. What they might do is try to protest publication of these results and stir up opposition in the business community and the Chamber of Commerce. And to get the painting manufacturers in high dudgeon about how they formulate their product."

"They can protest all they want," Merkel said, warming to the argument. "They simply can't prevent publishing our study. If it passes peer-review at a journal, it will be published. I promise that. That's what we do as scientists, not get intimidated by anyone, big manufacturers, or property owners, or demagogue politicians. We're talking about the health of kids and that's a helluva lot more important."

McDonough was quiet for a few moments, then said, "You know, this reminds me of a play. I'm sure you all remember it. It was set in the late 1800's and called 'An Enemy of the People' by the Norwegian playwright Henrik Ibsen. You know that play?"

Merkel and Crocker nodded. "I recall the play vaguely," Crocker said. "Remind me of the theme."

"It's about a Doctor Stockmann in a small community, who tried to call attention to the bacterially contaminated water supply in his brother's spa, an important business in the town's economy. The doctor's passionate and sometimes irrational anger and self-aggrandizing statements caused the town to turn against him. The 'enemy of the people' in the eponymous title. I'm not suggesting this situation is strictly analogous, but I couldn't help but think of that play."

"Yeah, I now remember that play, it's a classic, but the protagonist was his own worst enemy, as I recall," Merkel said. "But it was not about a scientific study, but only a letter to the local newspaper, many years ago in a different country," he said. "However, I get your meaning.

"My question is: What should we do now?"

"I wanted to meet so we are in conversation with one another," McDonough said. "This office is fully supportive of your work and your scientific publications. But I'd like to avoid escalation of the rhetoric. I can't, and wouldn't, prohibit you from doing it, but I'd prefer there be no more newspaper or television or radio interviews about this. I know Reverend Hightower helped you publicize the project on his radio show, and that was great, but I'd like us all to keep our heads down for now. Can we agree?"

"That's reasonable," Merkel said. "The Department of Public Health, the county and the state legislature have a lot to do to move this forward. My guess is that this will be a long haul and there'll be many slips between cup and the lip before new laws and regulations are in place. But we've provided an initial scientific basis for all that. And more research is needed to corroborate our findings. That all will take time. My only hope is that we can stem the tide of damage to children. One thing we can't control, however, is our community's reaction. So, we'll just have to wait and see about that."

Ben listened and admired how eloquent Dr. Merkel was. He was so much more than his reputation as a grump. His work in his own field of hematology was well-recognized internationally and his help in this project had been immense.

They left the meeting with Ben having mixed emotions. On one hand he was gratified that he had the support of admired colleagues and the legal department of the hospital. On the other hand, he was saddened by the mean-spiritedness of some forces in the society. He was eager to go home. This had been a long day already.

Chapter 39

Braxton Hicks

Ben pondered the discussion on his way home. He knew he wasn't a Dr. Stockmann from the Ibsen play, but he also knew his own passion and self-righteous attitude could get him into trouble if he didn't moderate his temper. Now he was absorbing the notion that his mission to rid the community of childhood lead poisoning was destined to take a long time.

First, he grudgingly acknowledged that more research was needed to confirm his teams' findings. Waking up the legislators to this problem and getting them to craft laws to combat it could take months, even years, to happen. In the meantime, the toxicology clinic's availability needed to be made well known to the community. More kids needed to be screened for lead and other toxic chemicals in their blood. Their homes needed somehow to be made safer.

The necessity of having a poison control center had long been discussed, but now the hospital administration recognized how essential it was for children's health. It could become a reality soon. But Ben finally realized this would all take time -- a lot of time. Ben's natural impatience with the pace of progress had to be tempered and finally, he knew it.

"I'm home!" he called out when he was helped up the stairs to their apartment by the restaurant guys. He looked at his watch and realized Cathy wouldn't be home yet from Channing. It was only four o'clock. He was so absorbed by the meeting he'd forgotten to return to his office.

"Hi Rosemary, it was late, and I decided not to come back to the office," Ben said when he called his office. "Any messages for me?

"I wondered where you were!" she said. "Cathy called. She thought she was in labor and went to the Lying In to be checked. She was admitted because they were concerned she might be. You should call the hospital," giving him the number.

With his heart pumping rapidly, he called the number.

"Nurse's station, third floor," came the reply.

"This is Dr. Ben Levinson," he said, breathing heavily. "My wife, Cathy, was admitted. I'm calling to find out how she's doing."

"Just a second, I'll let you talk to her nurse."

"Hello. Dr. Levinson? I'm Cathy's nurse, Josie. She's settled down. No more contractions. We think it was simply Braxton-Hicks. No bleeding. She's comfortable. Probably can go home later today."

Ben breathed out. He knew Braxton- Hicks contractions were simply false labor. "Can I see her?"

"Yes, come anytime. We have open visiting hours."

When he came into her room in his chair, she looked at him, then covered her eyes.

"I'm so embarrassed," she said. "I'm a nurse and should know better."

"Don't be silly. You're a human being, not a nurse, when it comes to your own body. I've been there. Now you know how it feels being on the other side of the doctor-patient relationship," Ben said, teasing her a bit. "How're you feeling?"

"Okay. I think they're gonna let me out this afternoon. Can you stay until I know and then take me home?"

"Oh, I don't know. I have some things I have to do," he said, looking out the window. "Of course, you silly goose, I'll stay and take you home."

They left with smiles a few hours later. On the way home, Ben asked the question.

"Your thoughts about the house?"

"I think we should buy it," Cathy said calmly. "It's not perfect, but we can improve it. Dad said he'll help."

"Good. I'll call Jocelyn and get the ball rolling. No telling when you're going to go into real labor. Good wakeup call."

"Yeah, that's the way I feel too. I'd like to get into that house before I deliver. It's fun to think about."

The next couple of months flew by as they got the house move-in ready. When Cathy did go into labor, they'd been in the house for three weeks and everything was in order. Ben had most of the assists he'd had at home. The new kitchen was completed in record time with Jack's help getting all the contractors lined up. Most importantly, the nursery was equipped and ready to welcome the new baby. They decided to wait to paint those walls with any color, though, until they knew what they had a boy or a girl.

Chapter 40

The Real Thing, June 1957

"Ben, my water just broke!" Cathy called from the bathroom. "Come right away."

Ben struggled out of bed, glanced at the clock -- seven -- got his braces attached, grabbed his crutches, swung into the bathroom. Cathy was toweling up the mess.

"Stop! That can wait. You having any contractions?"

"About every 8 minutes. Not too bad, but I'm surely in labor this time!"

"Go back to bed, or the chair, wherever you feel most comfortable. I'll get the car out of the garage. I don't think we need to go yet. This is your first baby, and labor takes a while. Remember all the stuff they told us in childbirth class? I'll try to remember, too," Ben said, reassuring himself as much as Cathy.

"Eat something, Ben. This could be a long day, and you get grouchy when you're hungry."

"Should I call your parents? Or mine?"

"Let's wait a little while until we get a sense of how long this may take. I don't want the whole family getting up in arms," Cathy said, much calmer than Ben. After all, she was from a large family, had seen this play before, and Ben was an only child.

The contractions got closer together as the day progressed, lasting longer, and becoming ever more uncomfortable. Cathy was a trouper and tried to minimize her experience so Ben wouldn't get overly excited. But when the contractions came every four minutes, she decided it was time to go. Between contractions she made her way to the garage and got into the Suburban. Ben did what he had to do to get into the driver's seat and they were off to the Boston Lying-In Hospital.

Ben pulled up to the emergency entrance and honked the horn, as he'd been told to do. A nurse came out with a wheelchair for Cathy, and she was whisked inside. Ben found the parking lot, went into his well-practiced routine, got out of the car, retrieved his wheelchair, and went into the hospital.

"My wife just came in, Cathy Levinson," he said, trying not to sound too nervous.

"Yes, she's up in the labor room, second floor. She's doing well, so don't worry. Can I help you find the elevator?"

"Yeah, that would be great. I'm fine once you point the way."

He could hear Cathy's moans as soon as he wheeled into the corridor of the labor unit. He hurried down the hall and a nurse knew who he was looking for. There was only one other woman in labor.

Cathy was sweating and straining when he walked in.

"She's about 80 percent dilated and effaced," the nurse said. "We're going to take her into the delivery room soon."

Between contractions, Ben kissed her, even though her eyes were closed as she tried to rest. He whispered encouragement and she nodded and squeezed his hand.

Dr. Cochran poked his head into the room.

"Hi Dr. Levinson. Things are going according to Hoyle. We're taking her into Delivery now."

"Can I come in too?"

"Sorry, not allowed. We're trying to change the rules about fathers being in the delivery room, but so far, we haven't been successful. I'll come out just as soon as she's delivered."

Ben considered arguing that he was a doctor, couldn't they make an exception, but by then the delivery was underway. In a short time, Dr. Cochran came out with a smile on his face and said, "Congratulations! You have a fine new son! Mother's doing well and laughing. They'll be out shortly."

When Cathy came out with the baby nestled in the crook of her left arm, Ben pulled his chair to the gurney, looked at his new baby, began to cry. Since he couldn't reach Cathy's face to kiss her, he grasped Cathy's hand, kissing it repeatedly and Cathy did the same to his hand. Later, when she was resting comfortably in her hospital room, they embraced and kissed in a more suitable way to honor the occasion.

"What do you want to name him?" Ben whispered.

"You have any ideas?"

"I have no idea."

"I wondered about Abraham. You adored your uncle."

Ben contemplated this, surprised he hadn't thought of it. Then he remembered that in Jewish culture, one didn't usually name a child after a living family member. But, of course, Abraham was not living. Anyway, Ben had already departed from strict Jewish culture by marrying his fabulous Cathy.

"It's not only my choice, my dear. Are you thinking about particular names? No old boyfriends, though," he laughed.

"Don't worry about that, none of my old boyfriends deserve it. I have a deal for you. You name this baby, and I'll name the next one. Hopefully a girl. Okay?"

"You sure? What if I wanted to name him Oswald or Leroy?"

"A deal's a deal. But I think you'll choose Abraham."

Ben went to the visitors' phone, called Jacob and Sophie, then Jack and Meg.

"We are now proud parents!" he shouted into the phone. "A six-pound, 13-ounce boy, black hair, perfectly formed, crying for food like his dad, and the docs say he's quite healthy. Cathy is feeling fine, but like all mothers who just delivered, a little tired."

Sophie and Meg cried, Jack gave out a whoop of joy, Jacob said "Well done! When can we see the baby?"

"Probably tomorrow. It's late now and I doubt they would allow visitors now."

"Have you picked out a name?" Sophie asked.

"We're thinking about Abraham," Ben said with some hesitation, never thinking until now that his father might be offended that he chose his uncle's name and not his.

"I like that," Sophie said. "I'm sure your father will too."

Jack and Meg also asked about a name and Ben realized how important naming is, especially to grandparents. He told them what they were thinking about, and their response was the same as Sophie's. The die was cast. Abraham Levinson.

When Ben came back into Cathy's room, Abraham was rooting around for Cathy's nipple as she smiled down at him.

"He's a greedy little guy," she laughed. "He's doing a good job, but it hurts a little. I guess I'll get used to it."

Ben looked at the two of them, mother and infant, and a warm feeling of tenderness came over him. He'd heard stories about the transformative experience of being a new parent right after birth, but he never realized, even as a pediatrician, how moved he would be by this. He'd carry this moment forward for the rest of his life.

"Adam? Ben. Cathy just delivered a boy, six pounds 13 ounces, perfect in every way. Both are doing well. What are you doing?"

"Wow, that's great! I'm home listening to a Red Sox game. A lot easier than what you're doing."

"But not nearly as satisfying. What an experience! I'll tell you about it when you come to see us and the new baby. We're naming him Abraham, after my uncle."

Ben's spirits soared to the ceiling, joining all the other fathers over the years in their joy at the Boston Lying In Hospital. He wheeled his chair down the hall, humming and smiling, with a tear rolling down his cheek.

Thirteen months later, Cathy delivered a little girl, seven pounds even, and Cathy, as agreed upon earlier with Ben, named her Jessica. When she brought Jessica home, Abraham looked at her curiously, wondering what this new creature was. But soon he toddled off, more interested in exploring his toys than his new sister.

Luckily for Abraham and Jessica, Ben had ensured the painted surfaces in their new home were all lead-free.

Chapter 41

Kennedy's Assassination, 1963

Adam's Book

"President Kennedy shot in Dallas!" came the announcement on the News Channel. "He's being taken to Parkland Memorial Hospital for treatment!"

"Kennedy pronounced dead at Parkland Hospital! Killer at large. Investigation ongoing. International and national conspiracies feared."

"Kennedy was shot as he rode in a convertible through Dealey Plaza. Governor Connally also wounded. Bullets came from high-powered rifle fired from window in Texas School Book Depository in Dallas shortly after noon today."

"Suspect of killing apprehended!"

"Name released of alleged assassin: Lee Harvey Oswald. More details forthcoming as information is made known."

The assassination of President John F. Kennedy was the most tumultuous world event since World War II. The shock everywhere in the world was unimaginable.

"I am stunned beyond belief," Ben said to Rosemary as he wheeled into his office after seeing a patient in the hospital. His secretary could only nod, still astounded and grief-stricken with this terrible news. She was so overcome that she couldn't even respond.

The most common question people asked each other in the days to come was "Where were you and what were you doing when you got the news of Kennedy's assassination?" Most everyone had that answer with complete and surreal clarity. That was certainly true with Ben.

"I was counselling a mother who had just delivered a baby with no arms," he told Cathy when he got home. "She'd taken thalidomide during the first few months of pregnancy for morning sickness."

Her case, and many others, prompted a plethora of studies on thalidomide's effect on the developing fetus. All studies concluded with the unequivocal finding that thalidomide caused these deformities. The drug was banned but too late for between the 10,000 and 20,000 children born with deformities, the worst of which was phocomelia -- foreshortened or missing limbs. The Federal Drug Administration had never approved the drug but the company making it had distributed it widely for "testing" anyway.

"How the distribution of this drug occurred without FDA approval is still a mystery to me. It emphasizes the importance of governmental regulatory agencies," Ben told Cathy.

"Where were you today when the news came?" Ben asked Cathy, who was still trembling hours later.

"Sitting at my desk when my secretary rushed in, crying hysterically, screaming that Kennedy was dead. I was incredulous at first but seeing her unravelling before my eyes prompted me to find a television. That did it. The same pictures, scrolling on the tube, over and over. The reports from all over the world coming in, all expressing horror that such a thing could have happened."

"Why is it that two of our most caring presidents -- Lincoln and Kennedy -- died by an assassin's bullet? What is it that makes goodness awaken such evil in the hearts of some men?" Ben mumbled into Cathy's ear as she sat on his lap for consolation.

"Have you talked to your folks?" Ben asked.

"No. Have you?"

"Haven't screwed up my courage," Ben replied. "They loved Kennedy. I ought to call them, and you should call your parents too. We've also got to figure out how to handle this with the kids. Luckily, they're too young to be as saddened by this as we are."

The next two days brought further after-shocks. Lee Harvey Oswald, a man, as it turned out, with a history of mental instability, was shot and killed by

Jack Ruby, a local night club operator, while Oswald was being transferred from the basement of a Dallas police station to the county jail. No one could understand how Ruby got into this area with a gun. The Dallas police never gave an adequate explanation.

This national and international trauma didn't go away for months. For many it never went away. Vice-President Lyndon Baines Johnson was immediately sworn in as President aboard Air Force 1, the presidential airplane, with Jackie Kennedy standing at his side as witness. Ben marveled at her strength in the face of this personal tragedy. Bobby Kennedy, the President's brother and close confidant was devastated and disappeared from the public eye for months. The reality of mortality was seared into many people's psyche for months, years, and for some, for the rest of their lives.

But the world went on, albeit with a heavier heart.

~~~

"Ben, got good news today! My book's almost ready for distribution!" Adam said as he sat down for lunch with Ben at Billy's. He could hardly contain his exhilaration. "It's 350 pages long and the proofs look wonderful. Great cover, too."

"Fantastic! What title did you end up choosing?" Ben knew he'd contemplated several titles, agonizing on the pros and cons of each.
~~~

"You know the concept of Occam's Razor? The simplest explanation is preferable to the more complex? I settled on "Child Abuse and Neglect: A Systems Approach.""

"You know what your fellow Marylander H.L. Mencken said? 'For every complex problem there is a solution that is simple, neat, and wrong,'" Ben teased. "But Mencken was a curmudgeon, so let's just ignore him."

"Easy for me. I never read his grouchy columns anyway. I like my title. It explains succinctly what the book's about."

"How did you find your publisher?" Ben asked.

"They found me. As you know, I'd published a bunch of articles in journals about child abuse. They contacted me and suggested I broaden the discipline from physical child abuse to include child sexual abuse, emotional abuse, and neglect, make it into a textbook. They argued that since all organs in the body can be involved in physical abuse, why not show how each organ system can be affected. Then by adding child neglect, which really makes up most of the cases of maltreatment, the book expanded. It worked for me, but it was a helluva lotta effort. I can't wait to see the final version."

"Me too. We ought to make a special section in our curriculum for abuse and neglect. Students need to know about this dark side of pediatrics."

"I already have a curriculum. Been working on it while I wrote the book. I'm ready whenever you are."

Ben was in charge of the curriculum for medical students and residents and was already expanding it to include topics in the new genre of "social pediatrics." The specialty of pediatrics was moving, although at a glacial pace, to emphasize non-hospitalized patients, the overwhelming majority of kids needing medical attention. Preventive pediatrics had been given a big boost from the polio vaccines and parents were now eager to get their kids protected by an expanding menu of vaccines. Also, the concept of vaccines opened their eyes to various other prevention strategies.

"How's the poison center effort going?" Adam asked.

"Comin' along. I'm meeting with a guy at the Boston Pediatric Hospital -- he's sort of the assistant to the chief there -- to move this ahead. He's very committed to the concept. Naturally he's hoping it will be sited at his hospital, but I think it doesn't matter where it is, only that it is."

So typical of Ben, Adam thought. Seldom thinks of who gets the credit, only that it helps kids.

"Heard anything new about the lead poisoning thing in the legislature?"

"Only that it's moving along. Making laws is not for the impatient. A new law must go through so many stages, pass so many reviews." He folded his hands across his chest and sighed. "Then there's the politics. As we learned from our dealings with the Public Health Commission, there's lots of opposition to any new law or regulation regarding private property. We're gonna have to wait until public opinion influences individual legislators to discern which way the public opinion wind is blowing before they commit to anything. Politicians have one thing at the top of their priority list -- the next election."

"Well, your publications on lead are making you well-known," Adam said. "And your review articles on common pediatric illnesses and vaccines. How many speaking engagements have you had?"

"Quite a few, I don't keep count. But there's a lot of interest not only locally, but all over the country."

"And your toxicology clinic is busy as hell. You're lucky to have a nurse who's knowledgeable and committed."

"Yeah, she really manages the whole thing. I'm lucky."

Changing the subject, Adam asked Ben, "How're the kids?"

"Both doing great. They're starting school next week, Abe in first grade, Jess in kindergarten."

"Public school in West Rox?"

"Well, no, not really," Ben said, a little sheepish that his liberal soul had been challenged when it involved his own kids. He had to admit they were going to a private school in Dedham, the next town over.

"We've enrolled them in Baron and Brownleigh. I know, I know," he apologized. "But there's been so much turmoil in the city's school system. Fights over curriculum, class size, all that stuff. So, we investigated it and decided that for us the best course was private school. Selfish maybe, but when it comes to the kids, we are selfish. We want the best education they can get. It puts a strain on our finances, but it's what we think is best."

Adam listened intently. "Don't worry about what I think," almost reading Ben's mind. "I agree with you. There's a whole lot wrong with the way public education is managed. It's not only the fault of the local school committees, who are grappling with a lot of fiscal and social problems, but with communities in general. A lot of conflicting priorities."

"So, what's new with you?" Ben asked.

"Got a new girlfriend."

"You sneaky devil! You didn't mention this when you were over for dinner the other night."

"Well, it's early, not sure where it's going yet. But promising."

"Wanna tell me about her?"

"Name's Susannah, she's about my age, a psychologist working with dyslexic kids at a special kids' school in Mattapan."

"How'd you meet her?"

"Met one Sunday morning at coffee hour at church, struck up a conversation and got interested in one another. We went out for dinner one night."

"And?"

"That's it. All I'm gonna say, nosey!" he laughed.

Ben joined in his laughter, and they headed back to the hospital. On the way Ben's wheelchair got blocked by a curb.

"Shit, I should know not to come this way. That damned curb is so high I can't get over it without help. There oughta be a law about making sidewalks and streets more accessible to disabled people!"

Adam helped him over the curb and said, "There's your next cause. Your plate's gonna be full of missions to change the world."

"A lot of changes are needed. Maybe I'll talk to my state rep about this. Like everything else, it'll take time, so we better get started."

"To change the subject, how's Cathy doing?" Adam said.

"She's so great. Now that both kids are going to school full time, she's going back to work," Ben said. "You know she has a PhD in public health. Now she's gonna use it. She'll be at the Margaret Conway Health Center as director of community outreach programs. That means she'll be promoting personal medical and mental health through exercise programs, good eating habits, vaccines, well child visits, and accident prevention. Other things too. I'm very proud of her.

And she's rarin' to go after spending the last five years at home with the little ones. She loved that, but her brain needs some adult contact."

"Yeah, Susannah says burnout is the most prevalent problem in special ed teachers. Mainly due to the lack of so-called normal adult interactions. We ought to get those two together."

Chapter 42

Up for Promotion, Summer 1966

"Dr. Friedman wants to see you sometime this week. When are you available?"

"Wednesdays are always my best days for meetings. What's this about?"

"He didn't say. How about Wednesday morning at eleven?"

"That's good."

"I'll get back to you. There's one other person I need to confirm for that time. Okay?"

Ben was trying to figure out what this could be about. The last time Friedman called was when they were jousting with the lawyer about the lead poisoning project. That all stopped as it waited on the legislative process that was still going on with no end in sight.

What could this be?

He thought about talking with Cathy about it, but decided he'd wait until he knew more.

When Wednesday morning came Ben wheeled down to Friedman's office. Who should he see there, but Adam?

"What are you doing here?" Ben said, totally confused. Friedman was not in the room.

"I could ask you the same question," Adam said, as he looked at Ben, completely flummoxed. "I have no idea why I'm here. You know?"

"Nope. What do you suppose we've done?"

"Beats me. Oh, here he comes."

Friedman walked in and without looking at Ben and Adam, took his place behind the desk, straightened a few papers, and then looked at them.

"I'm putting you both up for promotion to Associate Professor," he said, and then broke into a broad smile.

Ben looked at Adam who looked back, then they all burst out laughing.

"Good thing we're not cardiac risks!" Adam said.

"Or stroke. You trying to get rid of us?" Ben added.

"I knew you both could handle it," Friedman answered, "since you've both been through all kinds of stress in your relatively short professional careers.

"Congratulations, but of course, it's never a sure thing. You never know about promotions committees. They can get very picky, even testy, about promotions, especially above Assistant Professor. But I think you both are deserving of this. Each of you has published several important papers accepted by first rank journals, you've moved your chosen fields of interest forward, and you're recognized as outstanding teachers by students. Most of all, you're collegial and respectful in your interactions with other faculty."

Adam and Ben were dumbstruck and didn't know what to say. Finally, Adam blurted out, "When will we know?"

"Probably not for about six weeks. So don't schedule any celebrations just yet. I think your chances are excellent, but, as I said, one never knows." He paused, looked down.

"What?" Ben picked up on his hesitation.

"Well, there's one guy on that committee who worries me. He's from Mississippi and a bigot, I know that for sure. He makes racist jokes at departmental chairmen meetings. I think he also doesn't like me, don't know whether that means he's an anti-Semite too, but he's concerning. We'll have to keep our fingers crossed."

"Thanks for your confidence in nominating us," Ben said.

"I second that," said Adam.

They left Friedman's office quietly, but as soon as they were out of earshot, both gave up a whoop, shook hands, and embraced.

"What a surprise!" Adam said. "Can't wait to tell my folks."

"Sure was. And we both thought we were in trouble again!" Ben laughed. "That worry comes from a known fact: trouble comes often for people trying to make changes. Change is toxic, a person once told me."

Ben didn't wait long to tell Cathy.

"You want to kiss the new Associate Professor candidate?"

"Wow! When did that happen?" She dropped a dish as she was preparing dinner. Both kids looked up, startled by the clatter.

"Well, it really hasn't happened yet, I've only been nominated. So was Adam. Isn't that great?"

"Wonderful. You both deserve this. When will you know for sure?"

"Maybe six weeks. So don't tell anyone yet, especially the parents. But when it happens, we're gonna celebrate!

"How's that project you're doing?" Ben asked, changing the subject and focusing on her.

"Good things are happening. Got the okay to proceed with our 'HeadStart Roundup Day,'" Cathy said, with her characteristic understatement voice.

"This will ensure that kids in our health center are up to date with immunizations," she went on. "If they're not, we'll give them the shots they need on the spot. More than that, we'll have subspecialists there for consultations. For example, the ortho docs will look for scoliosis, gait disturbances, need for orthotics in their shoes. Stuff like that.

"There'll be cardiologists checking hearts, pulmonologists looking at breathing problems, especially in our asthma patients. Question and answer sessions about behavioral issues, developmental problems. The whole idea is to complement what goes on regularly in the clinic, but with more time, and it will give front line docs quick access to subspecialty evaluations. We'll be doing vision and hearing checkups, dermatologists will assess skin problems, special needs teachers will look for educational gaps. Really a great program."

"You know, we ought to do the same for our clinic kids. You say this is coordinated with, what is it, HeadStart?"

"Yeah, we got some funding from the new HeadStart program. In the catchy title of the program, the words run together with no space -- HeadStart."

"You always give me good ideas. I'll look into this HeadStart program. Where did that come from?"

"Part of Johnson's Great Society efforts. He's really run fast with a lot of terrific concepts, turning them into real programs, with real funding. I'm amazed at how much he's accomplished."

"Yeah, when Kennedy died everyone thought we were doomed. But Johnson's really been a juggernaut at getting things done."

Ben looked over at Abe and Jess who were fiddling with the rabbit ears on the television, trying to get the picture from rolling over.

"Put the ears up higher, maybe on the mantel. That might help," Ben said. It worked, with Cathy's assistance, much to Ben's surprise. This was one area in which he was not an expert.

"What are you trying to watch?" Ben asked.

"Flipper. He's a dolphin," Abe said.

"Sounds interesting. I'll have to watch it with you sometime. Sure it's a he?"

"I think so."

"I think Flipper's a girl!" Jessica protested.

"Look it up!" Ben said. "It could be either, but my guess is you'll not find an answer. But give it a try."

"Where should we look it up?" Abe asked.

"Good question. Maybe we should just write to the TV station and ask them. I'll help you find the address."

~~~

As Cathy and Ben were talking before falling asleep, Ben said, "I've been thinking about exercise lately. I don't get enough sitting in this wheelchair all day. I need to get outside more, not only for exercise, but just to smell the flowers and see squirrels and rabbits and butterflies. You know, what you and the kids see every day."

"And?"

"Well, maybe I need to go back to Arlene and ask her about what kind of exercises I ought to be doing."

"Good idea. You liked her. She still at the hospital?"

"Yeah, I see her from time to time. She works mostly on the inpatient services, so I don't see her that often."
~~~

Back at the hospital in the morning, Ben called Arlene's office, left a message, then went about his business. She called back later.

"Howdy stranger, how're you doin'?"

"Very well, thanks. How are you?"

"Still doing my thing. I hear about your exploits all the time."

"Hope you're hearing good stuff, not my terrible transgressions."

"If you're a bad boy it hasn't reached my innocent ears," she laughed. "So. What can I do for you?"

Ben told her what he thought he needed.

"Interesting you called. I was thinking about you just the other day.

"You know about the Boston Marathon, of course. The people who sponsor that race -- the Boston Athletic Association -- want to incorporate an event for disabled individuals -- wheelchair racing -- into the Boston Marathon. It's early, may not happen for a while, but I could find out about it and see how it's going."

"Please let me know what you find out. Is there a gym or someplace I could train to do this, what do you call it, wheelchair racing?"

"I'll find out and let you know."

"Thanks Arlene, once again, for your help."

A few days later she called Ben. "Got some info on wheelchair racing. This is catching on."

"Anything local going on?"

"Not yet. But that shouldn't deter you from beginning to train for future events. There's a gym across the street from the hospital, you know, where the swimming pool and the garage are. You could work out over there, getting your arms and shoulders developed further to move your wheels faster. They have a track around the top of the gym that people use for running. I bet they'd allow you to use that track to train on."

"Great idea! I'll call them. Thanks, Arlene."

In short order, Ben lined up times to train in the gym. This way he would have a goal for exercising. The gym director was very excited to offer this to Ben. He could envision a new mission for his facility.

After several months Ben had strengthened his biceps, triceps, and trapezius muscles. He was also now swimming regularly contributing to strengthening his upper body muscles. Cathy noticed his increasing bulkiness around the shoulders as well as his bigger appetite from all his exercise.

"I didn't realize when I married you that you'd turn into a Charles Atlas," she laughed one night as he polished off his third helping of pasta.

"I didn't know it either, but now that I'm into the body building exercises I can't stop. I've got to be ready when the Marathon committee finally allows a wheelchair division. I think they're getting closer to it."

"Do you have to get a special chair for a race like that?"

"I don't know, but Arlene told me the other day about a fellow in Cambridge who also had polio and is pressing the Boston Athletic Association to allow a wheelchair competition. He also designs special racing wheelchairs. Arlene told me this has been going on for several years at the Olympic games in Rome and Tokyo, so it's coming. Soon, I hope. I want to be ready."

"And I bet you're in it to win."

"Well, I'm sure if I'm in it there'll be others. Some of those others probably have been training for a lot longer than I. But just to do it, that's enough for me."

"Yeah, sure," she scoffed. "You're one of those strivers who always want to win."

Ben smiled, sort of embarrassed that she knew him so well. But glad she did.

"You're not a bad striver yourself," he said as he gave her a hug around her waist.

~~~

"Hey Adam, are you up for racing me?"

Adam looked at Ben, trying to figure out what crazy idea he had this time.

"Uh, sure. What the hell are you talking about?"

"Well, I've been training in the gym to run in a wheelchair race at the Boston Marathon. Now I'm so fit I figure I'm ready to challenge someone to a race, and since I'm friends with you, I thought you'd be a likely victim --- oh I should say candidate -- to race me."
~~~

"And where should this race take place? And who'll be there to declare me the winner?"

"I'll ask Cathy, and you can bring Susannah."

"Two unbiased referees, eh?"

"Well, okay, then, I'll ask my trainer to be the judge."

"Yeah, another unbiased person, right?"

"Who do you suggest, then?"

"Any other dude who happens to be at the gym when this momentous race occurs."

"Good idea. Let's set a date."

"So, when is the Boston Marathon race to be?" Adam asked.

"Well, not set yet. It may not happen for a year or two. But the Committee is working on it."

The arrangements were made, and all met in the gym. A fellow running on the treadmill was recruited to be the judge. And the race was on, with the wives yelling for their man to win.

Ben got off to the best start since he'd been practicing for weeks. Adam was surprised that Ben got up such a head of steam so quickly, so he had to match the effort. As they were rounding the first turn on the oval track, Ben cut ahead of Adam and took the lead. Soon, however, Adam got his adrenalin flowing and passed Ben on the final turn and won by several lengths.

"You cut me off on that turn!" Adam said when Ben wheeled up to him.

"Of course, that's part of the race strategy. Next time, though, I'll beat you. I know your game now."

"Oh, yeah? When do we have the next race? I can't wait!"

Cathy and Susannah came over, glanced at each other, as much as to say, "boys will be boys!"

"You two sound like a couple of adolescent males to us," Susannah said.

"Well, this is serious stuff!" argued Ben.

"Life is definitely a high school," Adam said.

Adam leaned over to Ben and whispered, "Great job, man. I'm proud of you. I'll go with you to the Marathon for sure."

"Thanks, friend."

Chapter 43

Disappointment and Redemption

Fall 1966

"Dr. Friedman's office called and wants you and Adam to come for a meeting," Rosemary announced to Ben when he wheeled into his office.

"Now what?" Ben said, then remembered he was a candidate for promotion.

"They never tell me. When can you go?"

They agreed on a time on Wednesday. He saw Adam heading into Friedman's office as he got there, so he assumed it was about the promotion. His heart began beating a little faster.

When they were all assembled, Dr. Friedman said, "I've got good news and bad news. The good news is that Ben has been promoted." Adam put out his hand for a handshake. Ben held back, fearing the worst. "And the bad news is that Adam was not."

"Was it the guy you were worried about?"

"We'll never know. Their deliberations are confidential. Listen, I'm going to appeal this. I'm really angry."

Adam sat quietly but Ben knew his blood pressure was going up.

"Well," Ben said, "I'm gonna reject mine. This is not fair. It's outrageous. Our professional accomplishments are almost identical." He was barely able to contain his anger, an old problem.

"My advice," Friedman said, "is to do nothing for the moment. As I said, I'm going to appeal this to the Dean. We've only begun this protest. Rejecting your promotion," looking at Ben, "won't correct this, so calm down with that idea."

Adam sat in sullen silence. It was almost as though he was occupying a different universe. Finally, he said, "Ben, please don't reject your promotion. That won't change things for me. It will change things for you, and it won't accomplish anything. I'll survive this disappointment. I've done so in the past."

"I've got to protest this some way. I'll think about it."

And that was it. The meeting was over. Ben and Adam walked out together. Neither knew what to say.

"How about coming to the house with Susannah for dinner tonight?"

"I'll find out if she's free tonight. I'll get back."

Disconsolate, Ben wheeled back to his office, called Cathy at her workplace, told her what happened and asked if they could have Adam and Susannah over for dinner that evening.

"I'm gonna be late tonight because of some things here I gotta do. Could we get takeout?"

"Sure. Pizza? Chinese?"

"Ask Adam and Susannah what they'd like. Anything's okay with me."

They settled on pizza and planned dinner for seven. Ben was not looking forward to discussing this huge disappointment, but he had to do this for his friend. What a shame, not only for Adam, but for the pediatric department and the medical school — and the city. A step backward.

But the evening was not all sackcloth and ashes. After they disposed of the raison d'etre for the dinner together, lubricated by some Gallo hearty burgundy, they laughed, cried, and embarrassed the kids. But good therapy.

It took six months to fix, but Dr. Friedman and other faculty members went to the dean, got his support, and the promotion recommendation was brought back. This time Adam's promotion was granted. When Ben and Adam met with Friedman, he told them.

"Was it that guy from Mississippi who put the kibosh on the promotion?" Ben asked.

"Well, no. It turns out that the real reason for the initial denial was due to a chemistry professor. He argued that studies done on clinical populations weren't 'true science' and consequently shouldn't qualify a faculty member for promotion."

"My promotion was granted, and I published clinical research. So, what's the difference between my research and Adam's?"

Adam was staring at Ben. "It's not the research," he said. They exchanged glances, both thinking the same thing.

"What happened then?"

"Some very heated argument. Several of us argued that we needed different criteria to promote those whose interests are in patient care and teaching. If we don't do that, we contended, we'll ultimately lose our best clinical faculty, who take care of our patients and teach our medical students, residents, and other health care providers. Their presence makes us an educational institution as well as one involved in bench research."

"I wish I'd been a fly on the wall at that meeting," Ben said. "I really hate academic snobbery. Snobbery of any kind, actually. So, how did the chemistry professor react?"

"He backed off and conceded he might have been too rigid. He dropped his objection. And the good thing is the committee is going to seek opinions from other academic centers about this issue of clinical versus basic science merit as it pertains to promotion. I think this was an essential discussion required for breaking down some hidebound attitudes that have divided us in academic medicine for decades."

As Ben and Adam left Dr. Friedman's office, Adam said, "I'm glad he's our chairman. He's a fair and honest guy who has his departmental colleagues' interests at heart."

"Agree. We're lucky to have him."

Chapter 44

Victory, 1971

"Dr. Levinson? This is Mary Agnew at the Department of Public Health. I've got some great news for you."

"Hi, Dr. Agnew. I'm all ears."

"The Massachusetts legislature just passed the Lead Poisoning Prevention and Control bill. Isn't that something?"

Ben sat there for a minute before the message got processed and absorbed.His mind returned to the early frustrations he'd felt when the hateful Dr. Eliot Zack, Commissioner of Health at the time, claimed there was no lead poisoning in Boston. Of course, that absurd claim prompted the studies that proved Zack wrong and saved countless children from brain damage and worse.

"Are you there?" Dr. Agnew asked.

"Oh, yeah, sorry. My mind was wandering. Finally, after all this time, I'm glad the lawmakers finally did their job. I've been watching and waiting for this news for months, even years! Thanks for calling to let me know. I'm very excited, ecstatic, to be honest. What a deal! What does the final bill do?"

"Among other things it requires property owners to control lead-based paint hazards in any housing unit in which a child under six years of age resides. That means the owners must make the paint unavailable to kids under six years old to ingest. It provides for enforcement by both a newly created state Childhood Lead Poisoning Prevention Program within the Department of Public Health and by local boards of health," Agnew said. "How do you like that?"

"So far, so good."

"In addition, the law enlists the help of the tort system for enforcement by providing that property owners would be liable for damages resulting from failure to make a child's apartment lead safe. And there are penalties for failure to comply. I'll get you a copy of the law when I get it."

"What a dream come true," Ben sighed. He paused before launching into his next stream of thoughts. "Mary, this is just the beginning. Now, we need to find a way to clean up the dirt around housing foundations where lead has leached out of exterior paint, get rid of tetraethyl lead in gasoline, ensure that lead batteries cannot be burned distributing toxic smoke into the air, and eliminate many other sources of lead," Ben rattled on. "You know, some toys are covered with lead-based paint. And that some pottery cups are coated with lead-based glaze that dissolves off in acidic beverages. So, this new law is just a start."

"So, how're you doing? I keep hearing good things about you," Mary said, and Ben could tell she was smiling.

"Don't believe anything you hear. But thanks for asking. I'm doing well. And you?"

"Very well. We're going to have a celebration with the sponsors of the bill in a few weeks. I'll be sure you're invited."

"Where will it be?"

"At the Statehouse."

Hope they have wheelchair access. That's one of my next projects -- making our disabled population have necessary ramps and elevators for all public spaces.

"You're becoming an urban legend. Keep up the good work."

"Thanks Mary. With people like you, we can make things better."

Ben hung up and moved his backside to a more comfortable position in his wheelchair.

There are many more challenges ahead. Finding out why kids die of sudden infant death syndrome. How to prevent it. Figure out ways to stop killing and wounding so many kids in our neighborhood. Why drugs are such a scourge. How to protect kids from violence and sexual molestation in their own home. Protecting women from domestic violence. How to spread Head Start programs all over communities. Shield kids from bad products that can injure or kill them.

Strengthen our schools, support our teachers. On and on it goes. So much to do, but we're making progress!

Uncle Abe, you watching from upstairs?

Epilogue

Ben raced in 1976 in the Boston Marathon, the second year. The man in Cambridge he'd gotten his wheelchair from—Bob Hall—had raced the year before, the first year it was offered to disabled persons. It turned out that the addition to the event was inspiring for contenders and spectators alike. Finding his calling—and succeeding at a new business—Hall made wheelchairs for many years for paraplegics.

At the end of Ben's illustrious career, in 2000, the pediatric outpatient department at Suffolk General Hospital was named "The Dr. Benjamin Levinson Ambulatory Services."

Author's Notes

Ben Levinson is a fictional character, inspired by Dr. Carl Weihl, University of Cincinnati Professor of Pediatrics and director of medical student pediatric education. Dr. Weihl was one of my pediatric professors during my studies at medical school. He taught from a wheelchair, due to his paralysis from polio.

Dr. Weihl taught hundreds of medical students in the art and science of pediatrics while overseeing the outpatient clinics at Cincinnati General Hospital and Children's Hospital Medical Center where the ambulatory services are named in his honor.

Since the early 1950s, when millions of people worldwide were afflicted with polio, vaccines, both Salk's and Sabin's, have nearly eliminated poliomyelitis everywhere. The Salk vaccine was made public in April 1955.

Initially there were complications with some batches of the vaccine in which the virus was defective causing several cases of polio. This fiasco turned into a bitter fight and litigation, but a properly manufactured vaccine was promptly administered to large numbers of kids with success well before the next polio season arrived. Hospital beds dedicated to polio patients decreased dramatically.

Smallpox is gone and measles, mumps and rubella are currently less frequent. But in 2024, immunization rates are lower than at any time in the past several years. Part of that is due missed vaccinations during the COVID pandemic, but also because of the drumbeat of misinformation about vaccines frightens parents into withholding proven vaccines from their children.

The International Stoke Mandeville Games Federation, or ISMGF, originated in 1948 when a man at Stoke Mandeville Hospital in England used wheelchair racing as a rehabilitation tool for injured veterans of World War II. The ISMGF teamed up with the International Olympic Committee and in 1960 held the first international games for disabled persons within the Olympics in Rome; in 1964, the name "Paralympics" was introduced at the games in Tokyo. In 1975, the Boston Marathon held the first of its annual wheelchair division races.

The Americans with Disabilities Act passed in 1990. Spearheaded by Senator Robert Dole, himself a disabled veteran, this law ensured access to public areas for millions of disabled citizens of the US. It would be expanded in future years.

References

Oshinsky, DM. *Polio: An American Story*. Oxford University Press. 2005.

Wunsch, H. *The Autumn Ghost. How the Battle Against a Polio Epidemic Revolutionized Modern Medical Care*. Greystone Books Ltd. Vancouver, Berkeley, London. 2023.

Allen, A. Vaccine. *The Controversial Story of Medicine's Greatest Lifesaver*. W.W. Norton and Company, New York, New York. 2007

Gittleman, S. *Reynolds, Raschi and Lopat: New York's Big Three and the Great Yankee Dynasty of 1949-1953*. McFarland & Company, Inc. Jefferson, North Carolina and London. 2007.

Drive-Master Total Mobility Center, Fairfield, New Jersey. www.drivemastermobility.com.

Reece, RM, Reed AJ, Clark, S, Angoff, R, Casey, KR, Challop RS, McCabe EA. "Elevated Blood Lead Levels and the in-Situ Analysis of Wall Paint by X-Ray Fluorescence." *Amer J Dis Child* 124:500-502,1972.

Reece RM and Christian CW. (Eds) *Child Abuse: Medical Diagnosis and Management*. Third Edition. Elk

Grove Village IL. American Academy of Pediatrics, 2008.

Kliegman RM, Stanton, BF, St. Geme III, JW, Schor Nina, Behrman, RE. (Eds) *Nelson Textbook of Pediatrics,* 22nd Edition, WB Saunders, Philadelphia, 2011.

Acknowledgments

My thanks go to many friends and colleagues who have been supportive and helpful in advising me along the way. My apologies to anyone I may have missed over the years of work on this manuscript.

Special thanks go to my writers' group, the Romeoriters—Salvatore Carbonetto, PhD, Jack Rosenbluth, MD, PhD, and Steve Treistman, PhD—whose professional lives were spent in scientific endeavors but whose lifelong interest has been in reading.

Thanks to my generous beta readers, Ed DeVos, Judy Singer, David Kerns, Jean Stern, Len Egan, and Jim Liljestrand, and to John Dowling, PhD, Arthur Silverstein, PhD, Hannah Wunsch, MD, MSc., Mike Tytell, PhD, Carl Heilman, MD, Newton Gresser, MD, Jaclyn Davin, OTR, CDRS, CDI, Rudolf Oldenbourg, PhD, and Barbara Struna of the Cape Cod Writers Center for their advice.

With much gratitude to Kathryn Galán of Wynnpix Productions, who led me through the maze of publishing with grace, steady and patient hands. And thanks also to Tom Tafuri for his excellent cover design and to Tom and Jenny Lutz of Impact Graphics, for creating the publishing covers.

Most importantly, a heartfelt thanks to Betsy Kyle Reece, for her editing, support, advice, and love.

About the Author

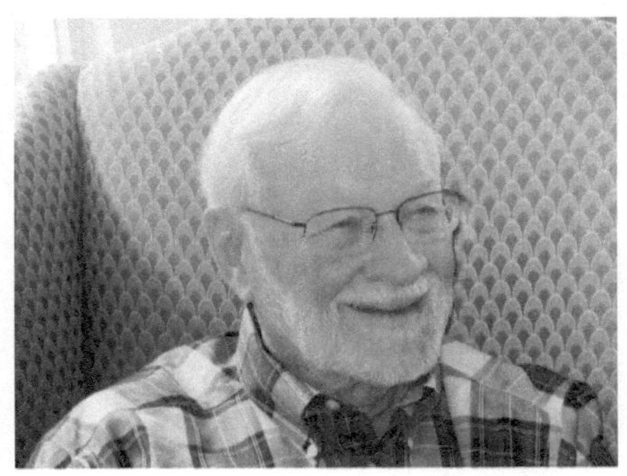

Robert M. Reece practiced, taught, and did research in pediatrics for over forty years, specializing in diagnosis and treatment of child abuse cases. He published nine textbooks, nearly fifty articles, and twenty-seven book chapters. He founded and was Editor of *The Quarterly Update* from 1993 until 2017.

His debut novel, *To Tell The Truth*, describes a fictional case of a young babysitter charged with the murder of a seven-month-old infant in her care.

In *Double Blind Double Cross*, he writes about surgeon Tom Barrett, a victim of post-traumatic stress disorder, (PTSD) and his experiences while participating in a clinical trial of a new drug for PTSD. Tom and two fellow patients immerse themselves in a high stakes investigation that reveals a shocking answer that would question practices in parts of the pharmaceutical industry.

In *Strong Medicine,* Dr. Barrett returns to shine a bright light on the pharmaceutical industry, uncovering practices that are unethical and illegal.

The Lewellyns from Vincennes is the story of a twentieth century family whose lives are buffeted by personal losses, two world wars, the Great Depression, and family triumphs. Based on a true story, its tapestry is woven with invention of scenes and fictional dialogue and is ultimately a tale of redemption and resilience.

Learn more at www.robertmreece.com